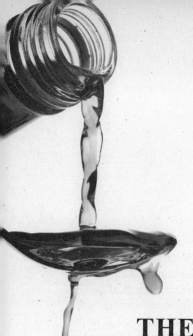

THE VINEGAR FORMULA GUIDE

By Emily Thacker

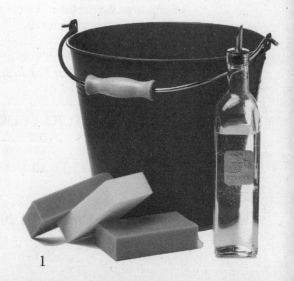

Published by:

James Direct Inc

500 S. Prospect Ave.

Hartville, Ohio 44632

U.S.A.

This book is intended as a record of folklore and historical solutions and is composed of tips, suggestions, and remembrances. It is sold with the understanding that the publisher is not engaged in rendering medical advice and does not intend this as a substitute for medical care by qualified professionals. No claims are intended as to the safety, or endorsing the effectiveness, of any of the remedies which have been included and the publisher cannot guarantee the accuracy or usefulness of individual remedies in this collection.

If you have a medical problem you should consult a physician.

ISBN: 978-1-62397-040-6

Printing 12 11 10 9 8 7 6 5 4 3 2

Third Edition   Copyright 2013   James Direct Inc

Table of Contents

A Personal Letter to My Dear Readers

Dear Valued Reader,

Welcome to the latest installment in my series of natural home health remedy books. I would like to first take a moment to personally thank you for sharing nearly 25 years of amazing remedies and health treatments that we have ventured into together. It is hard to believe that our discoveries together began more than 10 books ago, with the original publication of my first book, *The Vinegar Book*.

The Vinegar Book was the book that started it all, exploring hundreds of ways that a simple bottle of store bought vinegar could be used to transform the way we clean, eat, and particularly the way we treat both chronic and common health conditions and illnesses. Simple home remedies forever changed how we viewed both modern medicine, and the illnesses those medications were designed to treat.

The Vinegar Book has sold more than four million copies worldwide. It has been a journey of a lifetime, and I have been privileged to meet so many of you through your letters and emails over the years. (And now and then, I have been fortunate enough to meet some of you personally on my research travels.) Your ongoing letters have been a constant source of encouragement and inspiration to me. Hundreds of my readers have written to share their excitement about the multitude of ways vinegar has literally changed their lives.

In those letters, you have shared personal success stories telling of your own experiences with vinegar on everything from cleaning and sterilization, to health remedies and homemade tonics. (And more than once you have made me smile with a humorous tale or unusual anecdote for vinegar's use).

Also during this time, you have written with many excellent questions. It was with these questions in mind, along with others, that I finally decided to write this book. After more than two decades of research in converting vinegar concoctions and recipes that were passed down for generations into simplified formulas, and making tweaks and adjustments to each measurement to be sure it is just right for the job, I am pleased to bring you *The Vinegar Formula Guide*.

The Vinegar Formula Guide is a one-of-a-kind collection of exact formulas and measurements for all of your vinegar applications. In this unique publication, you will find step-by-step, easy-to-use instructions for your most asked questions concerning home remedies. You will find complete measurements for using vinegar both around the home and in the garden. And each listing comes in a user-friendly format for quick reading.

If you can read a recipe, you can use the formulas in this new book! What could be easier?

No longer will you need to wonder what type of vinegar is best for the job, or how much vinegar is safe to use. *The Vinegar Formula Guide* answers all of your most pressing questions.

As with all the research that goes into writing any of my home health books, my main consideration when bringing you natural health tips and remedies remains:

- Can this do you harm?
- Is it safe to use?
- Is it time tested?
- What does the research show?
- What are the benefits?
- What (if any) are the potential downfalls?
- What information is most helpful to the reader?
- How can I best convey this information?

I am confident that you will agree this research has brought you the most comprehensive publication to date on vinegar use in healing remedy situations and around the home.

As with any home remedy, or before making regular use of any natural health or alternative treatment, be sure talk openly with your personal healthcare practitioner about your plans prior to beginning a health regimen with vinegar. Keep in mind this book is an attempt to share information. And, as with any treatment, vinegar has its limitations. Be sure to use it wisely and always in moderation. Pay close attention to any warnings listed throughout the book, and heed all cautions presented by your healthcare physician.

Listen to your body. Remember to work hand-in-hand with your healthcare provider, and stay responsible for your personal health care needs.

So, let's get started delving into vinegar formulas together. I hope you enjoy reading *The Vinegar Formula Guide* as much as I have enjoyed putting this compilation together. I am hopeful that you will find the formulas beneficial and that this book will simplify putting the amazing attributes of vinegar to use in your everyday life.

Wishing you all my best,

Emily

PS. Looking for even more information on vinegar home remedies? Be sure and check out the back of this book. There, you will find additional information including publications on using vinegar as a home health aid and around the home. Plus, you can enjoy other home remedy books on topics such as honey, cinnamon, baking soda, garlic, tea and more!

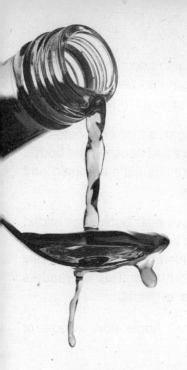

Chapter One

Introduction

As the latest addition to the James Direct, Inc. library of books on vinegar, perhaps you are wondering what makes this book different from others on the market. After all, this is certainly not the first book ever written on the subject of vinegar, even within our own publishing domain. You may have even come across other books about vinegar at your local brick and mortar, through an online bookseller, or on display in the checkout aisle at your neighborhood grocery store. So why another vinegar book? What could possibly be left to say?

Because we can confidently state there has never been a book written about vinegar like this ever before. It is not "just" another vinegar book, but a complete and concise reference manual for vinegar *everything*!

Vinegar has long been touted for its miraculous health benefits for the human body. Scientific research has verified that vinegar is packed with numerous vitamins and minerals, making it the clear choice as an all-natural, potent healer, and also an amazing household cleaning agent. Free from harsh chemical residues or unwanted medicinal side effects, vinegar has been used worldwide, throughout the ages, earning its name as "liquid gold."

Researchers have found that vinegar is not only helpful in lowering dangerous cholesterol numbers and boosting the body's immune system, but also can ease arthritis sufferer's pain and improve the body's circulation.

But at times, the research stated in vinegar books has ended up leaving almost as many questions as answers. While numerous vinegar home remedies have been written over the years, many of these helps were very general in information. This left readers with many excellent questions yet to be answered:

"What kind of vinegar is best to use? Apple cider vinegar or white vinegar?"

"Exactly how much vinegar should I use?"

"Can I substitute different types of vinegar?"

"What proportion vinegar to honey works best?"

This is where this amazing and unique book stands tall against all others. For the very first time, Emily Thacker, author of numerous popular home remedy books, makes available the complete *Vinegar Formula Guide*. This book is truly one-of-a-kind, providing exact formulas and measurements for all of your vinegar applications. No vague generalizations here. In this book, you will be introduced to step-by-step, easy-to-use instructions for better health, as well as for using vinegar around the home – for each and every listing.

The Vinegar Formula Guide provides a uniquely presented formula in a simple to understand format for each listing. No longer will you need to sift through paragraphs of information to determine the correct proportion of ingredients. This ground

8

breaking format takes all the guesswork out of using vinegar. You will no longer need to wonder, *"How much vinegar should I use to freshen my kitchen drain?"* You will not have to struggle with asking, *"Which is better to use to treat my varicose veins: apple cider vinegar or white vinegar?"* The Vinegar Formula Guide gives you concise and complete instructions for each home remedy and cleaning application.

This new books presents:

- What type of vinegar is best to use for each situation
- Exact formulas and measurements
- Step-by-step, simple instructions
- Indexed for quick reference
- Large, easy-to-read print
- Frequently Asked Questions section

This publication is not only a book, but also a reference manual for hundreds of the most fantastic and amazing uses for vinegar – many of which have never been addressed before!

Decades of research has gone into the making of this book. Untold hours of experimenting with different ratios and proportions help make this book one like no other. Our research studies have eliminated the need for guesswork. Now you can finally have access to real, working formulas to:

- Relieve nagging headaches
- Make your own daily health tonic
- Soothe painful corns and calluses
- End embarrassing dandruff
- Ease a sore throat
- Treat itchy athlete's foot
- Get rid of hiccups
- Prevent nighttime leg cramps
- Treat a sprained ankle
- End nausea

- Relieve discomfort of varicose veins
- Bring relief to arthritis sufferers
- Treat a tired or strained muscle
- Help heal and soothe itchy skin
- Treat swimmer's ear
- Have shiny, silky hair
- Fade age spots
- Settle an upset stomach
- Clean and freshen breath
- Soften hands
- And much more!

Some of the best qualities about using vinegar are that it is inexpensive to purchase and readily available – in fact, it is probably in your own kitchen pantry right now. And, because vinegar is all-natural, without harmful chemicals or dangerous additives, it is an obvious replacement for numerous health and remedy aids, beauty products and household cleaners. By using vinegar for your household cleaning chores, you eliminate the risks associated with chemical residues found in store bought cleaning products. You will find *The Vinegar Formula Guide* is packed with formulas for safe substitutions for store bought chemical cleaners for around the home projects, like:

- Clean plastic food containers
- Sanitize soiled laundry
- Give old floors new life
- Disinfect a bathroom
- Freshen a room
- Treat a garden
- Balance soil pH levels
- Clean brass to an amazing shine
- Get rid of mildew and soap scum
- Remove ugly carpet stains
- Freshen drains and septic systems
- Try a streak-free glass cleaner

- Revitalize and deodorize old drapes
- Remove tough ink stains
- Clean lead crystal and fine china
- Shine black kitchen appliances
- Make your own safe oven cleaner
- Clean and freshen coffee pots
- Remove rust stains from metal
- Keep bird baths clean
- Make an all-purpose spray cleaner
- Repel ants and other insects
- Eliminate pet odor and urine stains
- Make your own wallpaper paste
- And much more!

And, vinegar also comes free of the many side effects associated with today's prescription or over the counter pharmaceuticals. Vinegar is safe, completely natural, and full of life-enhancing nutrients.

Does that mean vinegar is a cure-all for every ailment in the body? Probably not. While vinegar's health attributes are well documented, and scientific research backs up many of vinegar's benefits to the body's immune system, no home remedy is perfect. And as with any health remedy, you will still want to consult your own personal health care provider before beginning a vinegar regimen. Also keep in mind that what works for one person, may not be as successful for another.

The Vinegar Formula Guide also covers a host of other often-asked questions surrounding vinegar and its use in the Frequently Asked Questions section in the back of this book. You will find answers to tough questions, such as:

- What is the difference between the two types of vinegar?
- Can I substitute apple cider vinegar for white vinegar?
- Can I make my own vinegar?

- Where can I purchase vinegar in bulk?
- How should I store vinegar?

Clearly, *The Vinegar Formula Guide* strives to make itself the complete guide for putting vinegar to use in the body and around the home. We hope you will find it your go-to reference manual for vinegar everything!

So, pour yourself a warm cup of tea, sit back and relax as you begin to delve into specific formulas for your vinegar needs. And don't be afraid to personalize these formulas to meet your own specific need or use. Grab a highlighting pen and a few sticky notes to mark a few of your favorite "must try" formulas. These formulas are intended to be as individual as you are. If you find you need a slightly stronger formula to clean away built up soap scum, for example, just add a little more vinegar. If you enjoy the taste of honey and want a bit more flavor in the elixir you have mixed to soothe your sore throat, by all means increase the sweetener. (See the section on "How to Use this Book" in the following chapter for additional suggestions on personalizing your copy of this book)

It is our sincere hope that this new format, filled with never before seen information, will allow you the greatest results in using vinegar as a home remedy or cleaning agent.

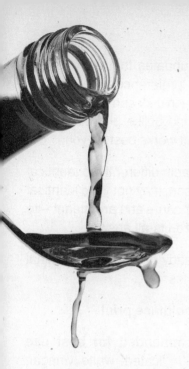

Chapter Two

How to Get the Most From This Book

This chapter is intended to help you get the most out of using *The Vinegar Formula Guide.* While this new format already makes using vinegar simple, we have a few additional suggestions that will help you get even more out of this book.

Do you remember the feeling you got when you purchased a brand new book, cracked it open, and tried your darnedest to keep its pages free from markings and in pristine condition? **This is NOT that book!**

This book is meant to be marked up, dog eared, highlighted, underlined, book marked and anything else you need to do to make it your own!

As stated in the Introduction, this book is truly like no other vinegar home remedy publication. Instead of ordinary reading or dry dictation, this book is meant to be completely personalized and the formulas adapted to your individual needs and circumstances.

This allows you, the reader, to make updates that benefit your particular lifestyle needs or personal preferences. This is the beauty of the world of home remedies. Each user can discover what works best for their particular needs, and unlike pharmaceutical medications, change and adapt it to what works best for you.

Everyone's body is different and reacts differently to identical stimuli. So, what works best for one person, may not yield identical results for another. But, home remedies can – and are meant – to be personalized. They are not a one-size-fits-all answer.

The Vinegar Formula Guide is already printed in an original format. Each vinegar application indicates:

❶ Name of vinegar application in boldface print

❷ Which type of vinegar is recommended for best use
One of three vinegar listings will be indicated: white vinegar, apple cider vinegar, or either type. If both vinegars appear to work equally as well on a particular task, "Either Type" will be listed, and it is up to you and your personal preference or availability to choose which vinegar you wish to use.

❸ Vinegar Formula
Exact measurements are listed to give you a great result. Feel free to change or adapt these measurements for personal use. If you feel your coffee pot seems to need more cleaning "punch," go ahead and increase the amount of vinegar for the job. (More about this later!)

❹ Step-by-Step Instructions
These simple steps will take you from beginning to end of each successful vinegar application.

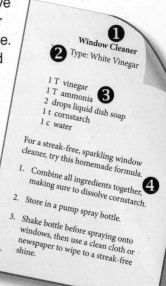

❶
Window Cleaner
❷ Type: White Vinegar

1 T vinegar
1 T ammonia
2 drops liquid dish soap
1 t cornstarch
1 c water **❸**

For a streak-free, sparkling window cleaner, try this homemade formula.

1. Combine all ingredients together, making sure to dissolve cornstarch. **❹**

2. Store in a pump spray bottle.

3. Shake bottle before spraying onto windows, then use a clean cloth or newspaper to wipe to a streak-free shine.

A Note About Multiple Formula Listings

In some cases, you may notice that there is more than one formula or remedy listed for a certain condition or use. This is not a misprint. Several successful remedies for the same malady have been recorded over time, each showing good success. It is up to you to determine which formula might work best for you.

One formula may use a flavoring. Another may use slightly more vinegar, or is taken more than once daily. Or, one formula may recommend an oral treatment, while the other is applied topically. This is an opportunity for you to discover which formula best meets your needs, taste preference and lifestyle. If one formula does not give you as much relief as you had hoped, feel free try another.

In addition, one formula may recommend an ingredient that you either find distasteful, or are already trying to limit or exclude from your diet. Some vinegar formulas include salt, for example. For those of you trying to eliminate sodium from your diet, you should be able to find an alternative remedy that does not contain salt.

So, how exactly can one personalize this copy of *The Vinegar Formula Guide*? Here are a few ideas to get you started:

• **Margin Writing**
  Use the margin area of this book to write any thoughts you might want to remember regarding how the remedy worked for you. You can also record any changes you have made to the formulas themselves to better adapt them to your situation and needs.

  You may also notice that one time of day works better for your vinegar home remedies than another. Perhaps taking a teaspoon or two of a homemade vinegar tonic right before bed works better than enjoying it after a meal. These are great notes to include in the margin area for future use.

- **Personalization**
  Keep a few of these handy supplies close at hand to help keep track of your favorite formulas and updates. Be sure and highlight a favorite or most often used formula for quick finding at a later date:

  - Highlighting pen
  - Sticky notes
  - Colored ink pens
  - Tab markers

- **Formula Changes**
  Feel free to change amounts or proportions of any formulas that you feel need adapted to you or your family's particular circumstances. While these formulas have been shown to work very effectively, personal preference plays a major role in home remedy adaptations.

  You should also be open to making substitutions, if necessary, as well. For example, many times one type of vinegar can be substituted for another without a noticeable difference in outcome. And, many of the formulas contain other ingredients which can also be changed or substituted for a variety of reasons. Which leads us to our next section:

- **Taste Considerations**
  Some formulas listed in this book contain additional elements to bring an added dimension of relief, or enhance palatability. These can easily be increased or decreased according to taste preferences without affecting the vinegar's potency. In some cases, you may wish to add an additional avenue of flavor to an oral recipe altogether. These can be added in the form of the actual product, such as honey, or in the form of a flavoring extract or oil. A few items you might consider adding :

  - Orange
  - Lemon

- Cinnamon
- Tea
- Honey
- Rose
- Fennel
- Ginger
- Cilantro
- Horseradish
- Red pepper
- Lemon
- Bay
- Anise

- **Length of Time**
Also keep cognizant of each application's recommended times and durations that are listed. As with other elements of the formula, these too can be altered according to need.

For example, while the formula may state to leave a vinegar solution on a mildewed shower curtain for 10 minutes, you may find that stubborn stains take longer to neutralize. Or, a poultice wrapped around a tired muscle may work fine, but you enjoy the feel or sensation. Feel free to adapt those times a bit longer if you feel you are benefitting from extended use.

- **Index**
Be sure and reference the index in the back of this book for quick referral for specific vinegar formulas. It will make searching for your favorite formulas faster.

A Word of Caution
Keep in mind that as with any product or remedy, different people and situations react uniquely. Be sure and test any fabric or other textiles in inconspicuous locations to make sure colors stay fast.

Prior to beginning a vinegar health regimen, be sure to consult your physician and talk about the pros and cons of the plan, in conjunction with any medications (prescription or over the counter) you might be taking. Also discuss any additional home remedies you are currently undergoing.

So, grab your highlighter and a note pen! It is time to get started discovering all there is to know about vinegar's amazing uses in *The Vinegar Formula Guide*.

Let's get started...

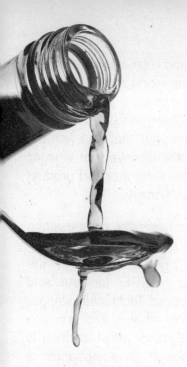

Chapter Three

What is Vinegar?

Before we delve into the first vinegar formulas, a little background on this amazing nutrient may be beneficial in putting it to good use.

What is Vinegar?

By definition, vinegar is a liquid that is made up of water and acetic acid. The acetic acid was formed during the oxidation-fermentation process of ethanol, which results in a liquid that contains between 4% and 8% acetic acid. Vinegar is a complex substance that is brimming with subtle flavors and aromas, packed with an assortment of nutrients, enzymes and trace elements.

For over ten millennia, vinegar has been one of the most useful and distributed liquids on the planet. Vinegar made its appearance 3,000 years before barley was grown to make beer, around 4,000 years before Mesopotamia was engulfed in a flood and approximately 5,000 years before the Egyptians learned to plow! Its versatility is virtually unmatched by any related formula. Vinegar's uses range from a flavor enhancing condiment to a cleaning agent for people, pets, and objects around the home. Countries and cultures around the world make use of its availability. When a sweet liquid, like grape or apple juice is sealed up and allowed to ferment, the sugar is changed to alcohol. If the fermentation process is applied a second time, this time with air, the alcohol turns to acetic acid. While the discovery of vinegar was probably accidental, it soon became such a prized product that mankind learned how to make it intentionally.

Vinegar is one of the oldest and most versatile compositions on the planet; but what is the chemical secret behind all its life-enhancing qualities? The English word "vinegar" comes from the French "vinaigre" – "VIN" for wine and "AIGRE" for sour. And that is exactly what it is: wine that has soured. Technically vinegar is a result of the oxidation-fermentation of ethanol. The resulting brew contains 4% to 8% acetic acid. Ethanol (ethyl alcohol) is converted to acetic acid (vinegar) through an acetobacter, a living substances that eats (oxidizes) the alcohol and produces acetic acid. Naturally produced vinegar not only has lots of acetic acid as a result of its chemical production, but the actions of the acetobacter infuse the composition with newly created enzymes.

The fermentation process is thought by some to have the unique ability to heal in addition to increasing nutritional values. Fermentation was originally an idea to keep food from rotting; however, the result can taste better than the original — just ask anyone who likes pickles.

The first person to develop vinegar however probably wasn't aware of its chemical composition and instead witnessed its revolutionary effects on day to day calamities. This new liquid was found to be an almost universal preservative and cure all. Food submerged in vinegar retained its flavor and color long after it should have spoiled. Festering sores, when doused with it, began to heal. Cooks in the kitchens of kings and doctors tending to the sick began to hail vinegar as an all natural cure all.

How is Vinegar Made?

Overflowing with complex flavors and aromas and laced with an assortment of nutrients, enzymes, and trace elements, chemically, vinegar is a complicated substance. The fusion of the sweet wooden storage barrels with the sharp, sour zing of the acetic acid creates the best tasting vinegar. Any plant that manufactures enough sugar to ferment into alcohol can become a parent to this substance. The distinctive flavor, aroma and healthfulness of vinegar is decided by the food from which it was made. The food then should have a pleasant flavor and aroma as these qualities will reflect in the finished product. Yeast is the key converter in the vinegar making process as its acetobacters cause the alcohol to change to acetic acid. Most scholars agree that vinegar probably started as wine that was exposed to oxygen in the air we breathe. Yeasts found naturally in the wine helped ferment it into what we now know is a type of vinegar.

Vinegar is made when a sugary liquid (such as pureed apples) is changed into an alcoholic one through a yeast reaction. Then, this chemical reaction is changed into an acetic acid containing solution. But vinegar is so much more.

Apple Cider Versus White Vinegar

Apple cider vinegar contains a healthy dose of pectin. This water-soluble fiber is easily dissolved in the body's digestive system, but remains in the body longer than insoluble fibers.

Apple cider vinegar is made from a wide variety whole apples that have been chopped or ground into smaller pieces. Sometimes apple peelings and cores are also used to make this vinegar. The different variety of apples used, sweet, tart, and even crab apples, help add to apple cider vinegar's full flavor and aroma. Cut apples are allowed to "breathe" for a period of time, allowing tannins to form as the apples react with air. This gives apple cider vinegar its rich color and flavor. The juice is then pressed or squeezed from the apples through a special press, and then allowed to ferment into a hard cider. These fermented apples give apple cider vinegar its aroma that it is noted for. As the hard cider then ferments even longer, vinegar is formed.

Apple cider vinegar is considered a very healthy, general purpose vinegar with a wide range of uses. It is an excellent choice for most pickling needs, cooking purposes and skin and hair care. It has a taste much like rice vinegar, and can be used interchangeably in recipes. Apple cider vinegar is notably packed with a storehouse of vitamins and minerals which are of enormous benefit to the human body. These nutrients can help restore a depleted body, or work to help bring its countless health benefits to those suffering from a multitude of conditions or ailments.

White vinegar is formed from corn which is distilled into corn alcohol. Additional ingredients are added to the corn alcohol and allowed to ferment into white vinegar. This fermentation process continues until all of the alcohol has left the product and only vinegar remains. Just like apple cider vinegar, white or distilled vinegar is completely natural.

Sometimes white vinegar can be manufactured from leftover products that are not only plentiful, but inexpensive. Since white vinegar is not made from the same source as apple cider vinegar, it lacks the distinctive aroma associated with fruited vinegars. White vinegar is also appropriate to use for pickling and for the preservation of foods. Because it lacks the deep color that apple cider vinegar boasts, white vinegar is a better choice for use on lighter colored foods and vegetables such as cauliflower or white onions. It also has less flavor to call its own, so it tends to interfere less with the flavoring of many delicate herbs.

This is considered one of the least expensive vinegars, so it is the best choice for cleaning projects, as the cheaper price allows for more liberal use. While most cleaning chores call for white vinegar, some food recipes use white as well. In most cases, the difference in vinegars is one of taste and volume, not so much effectiveness.

An additional reason one may choose white vinegar over apple cider vinegar is due to its lack of color. While apple cider vinegar contains many more nutrients than its white vinegar cousin, it can change the color of a light colored vegetable or delicate cloth. In these situations, some people prefer to switch to white vinegar.

Why is Vinegar so Good for Health?

Vinegar is a natural healing solution. Its unique medicinal properties are not only potent, but highly effective in preventing and eliminating the spread of illness, but also in promoting health and healing to already infected and ailing tissue.

Scientific research has shown that vinegar is rich in numerous vitamins and minerals the body craves for proper function. It is fat-free and contains less than 30 calories and only 2 milligrams of sodium in an entire cup. This makes it an obvious health choice for those watching caloric or sodium intake.

Scientists have discovered more than 90 different compounds or components in vinegar, most of which have enormous benefit to the human body. Substances found include:

- 33 Carbonyls
- 11 Alcohols
- 13 Phenols
- 8 Esters
- 7 Bases
- 7 Hydrocarbons
- 4 Acids
- 3 Furans

At one time, most researchers believed white vinegar did not contain much of the beneficial attributes that its close cousin possessed. But further testing revealed that white vinegar also contains a storehouse of essential nutrients. While apple cider vinegar still seems to possess a more potent health brew of these substances, white vinegar is now also revered as a health remedy.

A few of these essential health substances found in white vinegar include:

- Protein
- Calcium
- Phosphorus
- Iron
- Potassium
- Fiber
- Carbohydrates
- Vitamins A and D
- Folacin
- Zinc
- Niacin
- Magnesium
- Thiamin (vitamin B-1)
- Riboflavin (vitamin B-2)
- Ascorbic acid (vitamin C)

As for apple cider vinegar, the list of essential qualities is even more amazing. This vinegar boasts a list of healing compositions, such as:

- Vitamin A
- Vitamin B-6
- Folate
- Ascorbic acid (vitamin C)
- Thiamin
- Riboflavin
- Niacin
- Pantothenic acid
- Calcium
- Iron
- Magnesium
- Copper
- Zinc
- Potassium
- Phosphorus
- Manganese
- Tryptophan
- Isoleucine
- Threonine
- Leucine
- Lysine
- Methionine
- Cystine
- Tyrosine
- Valine
- Arginine
- Phenylalanine
- Histidine
- Alanine
- Aspartic acid
- Glutamic acid
- Glycine
- Proline
- Serine

Different vinegars, such as balsamic, wine, rice and champagne vinegars are derived from other sources before fermentation.

Each brings its own composition and qualities to the table. While these different sources can sometimes confuse scientists on why vinegar is such an amazing healing agent, they do agree that vinegar itself contains some very unusual properties that make it conducive to healing and healthier lifestyles.

Physicians know that humans need very tiny amounts of hundreds as of yet largely unidentified compounds. Scientific researchers in the field of nutrition are constantly discovering new minerals, enzymes, amino acids and other substances the body must have for complete health. Exactly how the human body uses many of these elements still eludes science. But, doctors do know that even a tiny deficiency of an essential health element can result in sickness, premature aging, or damage to brain tissue. The best advice today's scientists can give us to this point, is to eat a wide assortment of fresh foods, giving the body a wide spectrum of necessary nutrients.

Some believe that vinegar may be as close as we will ever come to a universal remedy for depleted nutrients in the human body. It also comes with a host of health-related attributes that are still being sorted out and cataloged. Many of these qualities can be game changers for someone who is dealing with health issues, or wishes to stave off some future health problems altogether.

How Do These Qualities Work for Better Health?

So how do these attributes actually work, and why are they important? Take a look at this list of vinegar qualities and what each has to offer. It is a pretty impressive list of health qualities that one would be hard pressed to find in another natural health substance:

Antiseptic

Infection preventer and fighter; prohibits the growth and spread of infections. Works to prevent the growth of illness-causing microorganisms in the body.

Antibiotic
Used in the prevention or fight of infectious disease; weakens and kills certain types of harmful bacteria and fungus.

Antibacterial
Kills bacteria or inhibits bacteria's spread or growth.

Anti-inflammatory
Can inhibit or prevent swelling an inflammation throughout the human body in places such as joints, muscle and other areas.

Antifungal
Kills the spread and growth of harmful fungus

Antiviral
Can kill or weaken harmful viruses; can also inhibit a viruses spread and stop a viruses growth.

Antioxidant
This substance that is found in vinegar's many vitamins works to inhibit oxidation within the human body. Antioxidants protect delicate cells within the body from dangerous free radicals known to promote many types of cancers.

Antimicrobial
Like the antiseptic quality mentioned above, antimicrobials work to inhibit the spread and potency of microorganisms, and even kill them altogether.

Each of these many substances works to not only promote better health and healing, but also to prevent many ailments and maladies from occurring in the first place. Whether you are using vinegar as an oral tonic, antiseptic medicinal solution, or to clean away germs and bacteria from your home, vinegar is an exceptional natural health solution that deserves consideration as a home remedy ingredient.

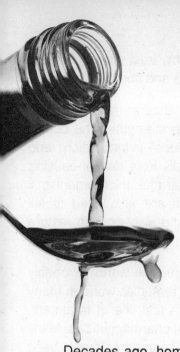

Chapter Four

Vinegar for Better Health

Decades ago, home remedies such as apple cider vinegar, were commonly recommended to treat conditions such as painful arthritis or gastrointestinal issues. Over time and with the advancements made in pharmaceutical medications (not to mention the astronomical amount of monies associated with the marketing and recommendation of these drugs), everyday home remedies were sent to the wayside in favor of new medications. But, as with many things throughout history, vinegar and other natural health remedies have come full circle.

One of the biggest reasons for vinegar's renewed appeal among natural health enthusiasts is that almost everyone has experienced the negative side effects of today's powerful medications at one time or another in their life.

Along with the benefits achieved by these medications, also came a host of unwanted side effects ranging from mildly irritating to downright worrisome. So, the field of natural health solutions began to gain new momentum. And vinegar found itself at the forefront of this movement once again.

People today, just as in days gone by, trust vinegar natural home remedies for many of their ailments and conditions.

The recipes and formulas in this chapter take the best qualities of vinegar and use that to help strengthen the body's undernourished immune system, reduce inflammation and swelling in the body, protect delicate cells from cancer-causing free radicals, and rid the body of harmful microorganisms. Vinegar's amazing antiseptic properties are also used to kill harmful bacteria in cuts and scrapes, and also work to restore vital enzymes to the body.

Will vinegar cure all the ills that plague the world? Probably not. But you may find that vinegar home remedies work on many common ailments and can be tried as a first line of treatment, oftentimes eliminating the need for potent pharmaceuticals. Many of the remedies in this book are the very same treatments used with success for generations to treat a host of conditions.

You may find that these vinegar remedies are highly successful in treating so many conditions you will want to use it as your first line of defense against health issues. Be certain to consult your primary care physician prior to making any change in your normal health regimen. And let your doctor know what medications you are taking, prescription and over the counter, as well as herbals and other home remedies.

In many cases, you will find more than one formula for the same condition. For example, several listings for formulas can be found under the heading of "Arthritis." This is due to the fact that many very successful recipes have been handed down for generations, with slight variances in ingredients. One remedy may work better than another, so if one is unsuccessful, be sure and experiment with another listing.

And remember, many of these formulas may require the benefit of time to begin working. While a formula to ease an upset stomach may work right away, oral concoctions for arthritis relief may need a couple of weeks to build up for relief. For instances like this, you may wish to try a topical formula in conjunction with the oral formula for immediate relief while you are waiting for the oral to take effect.

Now, let's explore these formulas together, and see what vinegar home remedies might do for you!

Arthritis Relief
(Apple Cider Vinegar)

1 teaspoon vinegar
1 teaspoon honey
1 cup warm water

1. Combine vinegar and honey is a teacup or glass.

2. Add warm water and stir until incorporated.

3. Drink a glass of this concoction in the morning, and another at nighttime before bed.

Arthritis
(Apple Cider Vinegar)

1 cup vinegar
1/2 cup honey
1/2 cup blueberries
1/2 cup raspberries
1 teaspoon lemon juice

1. Combine all ingredients in a blender.

2. Take 2-3 tablespoons each day to bring relief from arthritis.

Arthritis Relief
(Apple Cider Vinegar)

1 tablespoon vinegar
1/2 grapefruit
1 orange
1 lemon
2 stalks of celery
4 cups water
1 tablespoon of salt

1. Cut the celery, orange, grapefruit and lemon into chunks. It is okay to include the peelings.

2. Simmer uncovered in water for one hour

3. Press the softened ingredients thru a jelly bag or tight sieve. Stir in vinegar and salt.

4. When ready to use, combine 1/4 cup of this mixture into a full glass of water.

5. Drink one glass in the morning and evening.

Arthritis Poultice
(Apple Cider Vinegar)

2 egg whites
1/2 cup turpentine
1/2 cup vinegar
1/4 cup olive oil

1. Combine all ingredients in a blow or small tub.

2. Use mixture to massage into joints with a soft cloth for gentle relief.

3. Do Not Ingest.

4. If desired, turpentine may be left out of formula.

Arthritis Tonic
(Apple Cider Vinegar)

2 teaspoons vinegar
8 ounce glass of water

1. Combine vinegar and water in a tall glass.

2. Drink this combination before each meal, three times a day.

Headache Relief
(Apple Cider Vinegar)

1 cup vinegar
1 cup water
towel

1. Combine vinegar and water on the stove and bring to a boil.

2. Pour into a bowl and place on table.

3. Cover head with towel, over bowl, and allow vapors to rise; breathe these vapors for 5 – 10 minutes to bring relief from headache.

Headache Relief
(Either Type)

1/4 cup vinegar
water in vaporizer

1. Add vinegar to vaporizer water.

2. Inhale for 5 minutes.

3. Lay in a dark, quiet room for 20 minutes to bring headache relief.

Headaches from Elevated Blood Pressure
(Apple Cider Vinegar)

This remedy is rooted in Chinese medicine.

2 cups vinegar
2 celery stalks, cut in half

1. On the stove top, boil celery stalks in vinegar.

2. Boil for 5 minutes.

3. Remove from heat and allow to cool completely.

4. At first sign of a headache, chew on a vinegar fortified celery stalk to bring relief.

Stomach Nausea Relief
(Apple Cider Vinegar)

1 tablespoon vinegar
1 tablespoon honey
12 ounce glass of warm water

1. Combine all ingredients in a drinking glass.

2. Slowly drink mixture to bring relief of upset stomach or nausea.

Stomach: Indigestion
(Apple Cider Vinegar)

2 cups vinegar
1 teaspoon fresh ginger root, grated
2 teaspoons honey

1. Combine all three ingredients together.

2. Sip after a meal that has left you with indigestion.

Stomach Discomfort or Nausea Poultice
(Apple Cider Vinegar)

1/4 cup vinegar
clean cloth

1. Gently warm vinegar on stove top or microwave.

2. Soak clean cloth in warm vinegar, and wring out excess moisture.

3. Place warm vinegar cloth on stomach.

4. Can replace with new cloth once original cools.

Stomach: Digestion Problems
(Apple Cider Vinegar)

1/2 cup vinegar
1/4 cup water
1 teaspoon fennel seeds

1. Combine all ingredients and warm over medium heat to infuse fennel seeds.

2. Pour into a teacup and enjoy.

3. Add dollop of honey, if desired for sweeter taste.

Stomach: Heartburn
(Apple Cider Vinegar)

2 teaspoons vinegar
6 ounces water

1. Combine vinegar and water in a glass.

2. Drink this mixture about 10 minutes before a meal to prevent heartburn.

Leg Cramps
(Apple Cider Vinegar)

1 teaspoon vinegar
1 teaspoon honey
1 tablespoon calcium lactate
6 ounces warm water

1. Combine all ingredients in a drinking glass.

2. Drink entire solution once a day.

Muscle Aches
(Apple Cider Vinegar)

1/4 cup vinegar
2 wintergreen sprigs
soft, clean cloth

1. Combine vinegar and sprigs together.

2. Soak clean cloth in vinegar solution.

3. Apply to sore muscles for 10 minutes.

4. Repeat as often as needed.

Muscle Aches or Sprains
(Apple Cider Vinegar)

1/2 cup vinegar
1/4 teaspoon cayenne pepper
soft, clean cloth

1. Combine vinegar and pepper in a dish.

2. Soak cloth and wring out any dripping moisture.

3. Apply to sore muscle area for 3 to 5 minutes, 3 times a day.

Sprains
(Apple Cider Vinegar)

1 cup vinegar
Bucket of hot water

1. For muscle sprains that require a hot soak, fill clean bucket of with hot water (but not scalding).

2. Add a cup of vinegar to lessen the intensity of the heat.

3. Soak affected area for 10 minutes on, and 10 minutes off.

Feet: Aching Feet
(Apple Cider Vinegar)

1/2 cup vinegar
ankle-deep warm bath water

1. Add vinegar to warm bath water or to foot spa machine.

2. Being careful not to slip, walk back and forth in vinegared bath water.

3. If slipping is a concern, sit on edge of tub or in a bath chair and soak feet, moving them around as much as possible.

4. Rub vinegar water around joints and massage into feet and ankle area while soaking; be sure to press into the balls of the feet for added comfort relief.

5. Soak 2-3 times a day, as needed.

6. Dry feet when finished.

Athlete's Foot
(Apple Cider Vinegar)

1/4 cup vinegar
1 1/4 cup water

1. Combine vinegar and water together.

2. Soak socks in this mixture for 30 minutes.

3. Wash and dry socks as usual.

Shingles
(Apple Cider Vinegar)

3 tablespoons vinegar
2 tablespoons cornstarch

1. Combine vinegar and cornstarch to form paste.

2. Gently use paste to coat painful shingles lesions.

3. Keep on lesions and allow to dry.

4. When needed, gently rinse.

5. Apply as often as it gives relief.

Shingles
(Apple Cider Vinegar)

Vinegar, undiluted

1. Using a clean cloth, saturate with vinegar and then wring out most of excess moisture.

2. Place cloth over shingles for cool relief.

3. Once used, be sure and wash cloth in hot water to sanitize completely.

Skin Irritations: Welts and Hives
(Either Type)

1 tablespoon vinegar
1 tablespoon cornstarch

1. Blend vinegar with cornstarch into a thick paste.

2. Pat paste onto itchy area and allow to dry.

3. Gently wash paste off with warm water, followed by a cool rinse.

Skin Irritation: Boils
(Apple Cider Vinegar)

1 cup vinegar
1/4 cup fresh willow twigs, broken
clean, soft cloth

1. Simmer vinegar and fresh willow twigs on low heat until twigs are tender.

2. Use liquid to coat a soft cloth and use as a poultice on tender skin boils.

Skin Irritation: Eczema
(Apple Cider Vinegar)

2 teaspoons vinegar
1 teaspoon honey
8 ounce water

1. Add vinegar and honey to glass of water.

2. Consume this mixture 2-3 times a day for one week.

Varicose Veins Poultice
(Apple Cider Vinegar)

1/4 cup vinegar
clean cloth

1. Soak cloth with vinegar until wet, and wring out any dripping moisture.

2. Wrap leg with cloth.

3. Sit with leg propped up for 30 minutes, two times a day (once in morning and once in the evening).

4. Relief from pain should be noticed within 6 weeks.

Varicose Veins
(Apple Cider Vinegar)

1 teaspoon vinegar
1 teaspoon honey
8 ounce glass of warm water

1. Combine all ingredients in a drinking glass.

2. Drink once or twice daily; once after each treatment using above formula for Varicose Veins poultice.

Vinegar Daily Tonic
(Apple Cider Vinegar)

1 tablespoon vinegar
8 ounce glass of water

1. Combine vinegar with water.

2. Drink this blend daily for better overall health.

Vinegar Daily Tonic
(Apple Cider Vinegar)

1 teaspoon vinegar
1 teaspoon honey
8 ounce glass of water

3. Combine vinegar and honey with water.

4. Drink this concoction 3 times a day, 1/2 hour before meals.

Vinegar Daily Tonic
(Apple Cider Vinegar)

2 tablespoons vinegar
1 teaspoon honey
1 cup warm water

5. Combine vinegar and honey with water.

6. Drink this mixture, very slowly, before meals.

Influenza/Flu
(Apple Cider Vinegar)

Recommended by researchers at the Chinese Academy of Medical Science to kill germs that cause influenza/flu.

2-4 cups vinegar

1. Bring vinegar to a boil over medium heat.

2. Continue boiling vinegar uncovered, allowing vapors to permeate the room.

3. After most of the vinegar has evaporated, use remains to wipe countertops and door knobs.

Seasonal Allergies
(Apple Cider Vinegar)

1 tablespoon vinegar
2 teaspoons honey
8 ounces water

1. Combine vinegar and honey in a glass of water.

2. Drink once in the morning, and once in the evening for allergy relief all season long.

Nosebleeds
(Apple Cider Vinegar)

2 teaspoons vinegar
6 ounces water

1. Combine vinegar and water in a glass.

2. Drink this vinegar and water solution once a day to prevent nosebleeds.

Nasal Congestion
(Apple Cider Vinegar)

1 cup vinegar
1 cup water

1. Combine vinegar and water in a saucepan and place on stove top; bring to a boil.

2. Pour vinegar solution into a bowl and place on table.

3. Cover head with towel, over bowl, and breathe in vapors to help clean nasal decongestion.

Congestion
(Apple Cider Vinegar)

1 cup vinegar
1 – 2 tablespoons honey
1 clove mashed garlic
small pinch of cayenne pepper

1. Combine all ingredients in a small bowl.

2. Sip gently throughout the day to ease troubled breathing.

Sore Throat
(Apple Cider Vinegar)

1/4 cup vinegar
1/4 cup honey

1. Combine vinegar and honey together.

2. Take one tablespoon of this mixture every 4 hours, more often if needed.

Sore Throat
(Apple Cider Vinegar)

1/2 cup vinegar
1/2 cup water
1 teaspoon cayenne pepper
3 tablespoons honey

1. Combine all ingredients together in a glass or cup.

2. Sip on this homemade syrup concoction occasionally throughout the day, as needed, for relief of sore throat pain.

Sore Throat Gargle
(Apple Cider Vinegar)

1/4 cup vinegar
8 ounces warm water

1. Combine ingredients in a glass.

2. Gargle as often as needed at the first notice of a sore throat.

Cough
(Apple Cider Vinegar)

1 tablespoon vinegar
Clean pillowcase

1. Sprinkle vinegar over clean pillowcase and allow to air dry.

2. Use at bedtime to help soothe a dry, winter cough.

Cough
(Apple Cider Vinegar)

1 cup vinegar
1 – 2 tablespoons honey
1 clove mashed garlic

1. Combine all ingredients in a small bowl.

2. Sip gently throughout the day to ease a nagging cough.

3. Warm this syrup, if preferred.

Pneumonia
(Apple Cider Vinegar)

2 cups vinegar

1. Place vinegar in small pan and bring to a boil on stove top over medium heat.

2. Continue boiling vinegar uncovered, allowing vapors to permeate the room.

3. Repeat throughout the day, as needed.

Insomnia
(Apple Cider Vinegar)

1 tablespoon vinegar
3/4 cup honey

1. Prepare this vinegar and honey combination ahead of time.

2. About 20 minutes before bedtime, consume 1 teaspoon of this mixture.

Hiccup Relief
(Apple Cider Vinegar)

1 teaspoon vinegar
1 cup warm water

1. Combine vinegar and water in a small glass.

2. Sip mixture, drinking very slowly, until hiccups disappear.

Bladder Infection
(Apple Cider Vinegar)

1 tablespoon vinegar
8 ounces water

1. Combine vinegar and water in a glass.

2. Drink 2-3 times daily end bladder infection.

Urinary Tract
(Apple Cider Vinegar)

1 teaspoon vinegar

1. Take one teaspoon of vinegar every day for better urinary tract health.

Insect Bites
(Apple Cider Vinegar)

vinegar, undiluted
cotton balls

1. Dab vinegar-soaked cotton balls onto insect bites and stings to neutralize itching and pain.

Diabetes
(Apple Cider Vinegar)

2 tablespoons vinegar
1/8 teaspoon salt
8 ounces of water

1. Combine vinegar and salt in glass of water.

2. Drink twice a day.

Asthma Acupressure
(Apple Cider Vinegar)

1/4 cup vinegar
clean gauze pads
rubber bands

1. Soak gauze pads in vinegar until soaked through; wring out most of the excess moisture, but still allow pads to remain wet.

2. Use rubber bands to secure vinegar pads to inside of wrists. Do not allow bands to become too tight.

3. Repeat as often as necessary for relief from asthma symptoms.

Weight Loss
(Apple Cider Vinegar)

1 teaspoon vinegar
8 ounces of warm water

1. Stir vinegar into glass of warm water.

2. Drink full glass of vinegar – water solution 10 – 20 minutes before each meal to moderate an over-robust appetite and stimulate weight loss.

High Blood Pressure
(Apple Cider Vinegar)

1 teaspoon vinegar

1. It has been said that consuming a teaspoon of vinegar daily may help lower blood pressure.

Ear Infection
(Apple Cider Vinegar)

1 teaspoon vinegar, undiluted

1. Tilt head to the side, with ear facing upright.

2. Pour vinegar into ear canal, making sure solution flows all the way down to the infection.

3. Allow to sit for 30 seconds.

4. Tip ear to drain vinegar onto a paper towel.

5. Repeat three times a day, until infection is gone.

Ear Infection Prevention
(White Vinegar)

Prevent water-borne infections from settling in the ears. Great for use after swimming in a lake or pond.

3 tablespoons vinegar
3 tablespoons rubbing alcohol

1. Combine both ingredients together.

2. Using an eye dropper, gently rinse out ear canal to free any lingering bacteria.

Cholesterol
(Apple Cider Vinegar)

1 tablespoon vinegar
1 teaspoon honey

1. Each morning, consume a spoonful of vinegar and honey to help bring down cholesterol levels.

Cholesterol
(Apple Cider Vinegar)

Pectin, found in apples, slows food absorption in the intestines, allowing it to bind to cholesterol.

1 cup vinegar
2 cups chopped apples
1/2 cup honey
1/2 teaspoon cinnamon
1/2 teaspoon nutmeg

1. In a blender, place apples and blend with other ingredients.

2. Sip a few teaspoons of this fortified vinegar throughout the day, or serve over fresh fruit.

Diarrhea
(Apple Cider Vinegar)

2 tablespoons vinegar
1 teaspoon honey
8 ounces water

1. Add vinegar and honey to glass of water.

2. Drink 3 – 4 times a day until diarrhea subsides.

Diarrhea
(Apple Cider Vinegar)

1 teaspoon vinegar
8 ounces water

1. Add vinegar to glass of water.

2. Drink this mixture 4-6 times a day; formula will also help with avoid dehydration.

Constipation
(Apple Cider Vinegar)

2 tablespoons vinegar
1 teaspoon lemon juice
8 ounces water

1. Add vinegar to glass of water.

2. Drink three times daily.

Light-headedness
(Apple Cider Vinegar)

2 tablespoon vinegar
2 tablespoon honey
8 ounces water

1. Combine vinegar and honey in a glass of water.

2. Drink this mixture slowly, three times a day.

Food Poisoning Prevention
(Apple Cider Vinegar)

Some doctors recommend this formula when eating from questionable sources in foreign countries. This tonic should be used for the entire travel period as a preventative measure. Honey can also be added if flavor needs to be altered for a more palatable effect.

1 tablespoon vinegar
beverage such as vegetable juice or water

1. Combine vinegar with other desired beverage (stream or tap water is not recommended).

2. Drink daily as a preventative measure 30 minutes before meals.

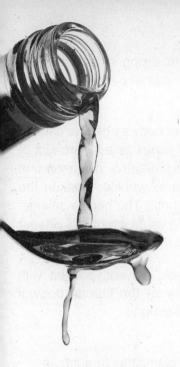

Chapter Five

Vinegar, Skin Deep

Vinegar's use as a beauty agent goes back as far as vinegar itself. Cleopatra was known to have trusted in vinegar. Ancient history is rich with chronicles detailing vinegar's place as a natural beauty agent.

Royalty included vinegar in the beauty regimen of princesses and queens. Women kept aged vinegar as part of their dowry. Ladies from all walks of life coveted the benefits vinegar was thought to possess in their search for an eternal fountain of youth.

While vinegar may not actually turn back the hands of time, there is scientific evidence to support claims that vinegar does have significant benefit to not only bring better health to the human body, but also bring cosmetic improvements to skin and hair.

Apple cider vinegar has been shown to help balance pH levels in the body. Vinegar's own pH is nearly the same of that of healthy human skin tissue, making it an obvious choice to right chemical imbalances. It is also an excellent natural choice for bestowing smooth, younger looking skin to the body, and can work to restore elasticity to damaged hair and promote strong shiny hair – all without the use of harsh chemicals that can deplete hair follicles and hair shafts of essential nutrients.

Science has shown that much of the body's aging is caused by free radicals. Free radicals naturally occur as a by-product of metabolism and are responsible for degenerative diseases that come with aging. They cause the skin to wrinkle, weaken the immune system and can accelerate arthritis. The body's defense against these free radicals are antioxidants. Much of the vinegar in this chapter can be used to help fight these free radicals.

Vinegar is an amazing water-soluble solvent, packed with vitamins, minerals and other essentials for the human body. It stands alone as a natural beauty aid, helping to:

- Restore youthful skin
- Combat pimples and other skin blemishes through its antiseptic properties
- Balance pH levels in the skin
- Deodorize naturally
- Strengthen and add luster to damaged hair
- Clean and open skin pores
- Soothe dry or damaged skin

While vinegar stands alone in its ability is to enhance and combat common skin problems, it can be taken to even higher levels when used in conjunction with other common household substances. Some of those most recommended items you will find used in the formulas in this chapter:

- Olive oil
- Baking soda
- Lemon juice
- Milk
- Granulated sugar
- Onion
- Petroleum jelly
- Tea
- Cornstarch
- Fresh and dried herbs
- Honey
- Oatmeal

Over the years, vinegar has been credited with the power to act as a soothing skin tonic, add beautiful highlights to hair, and bring a calming comfort or energizing feel to the bath. Vinegar is a natural solution that people have been using for hundreds of years to make people feel better. It can bring relief from many discomforts and is hailed for its fresh, pleasing aroma.

So, as we enter this new chapter, be prepared to learn new ways vinegar can work to keep you looking as young and beautiful on the outside, as your new found healthiness on the inside. All you need is an open mind – and a bit of vinegar!

Hair: Dandruff
(Apple Cider Vinegar)

2 teaspoons vinegar
1/4 cup water
comb or brush

1. Combine vinegar and water in a glass or bowl.

2. Wet comb or brush in vinegar solution and brush through hair, especially to the roots.

3. Rub remaining vinegar solution into scalp.

4. Allow to set 10 minutes and wash hair as usual.

Hair: Dandruff
(Apple Cider Vinegar)

1/2 cup vinegar
2 cups warm water

1. Combine vinegar and water in a cup or bowl.

2. Immediately after shampooing hair, rinse with vinegar mixture.

Hair: Dandruff
(Apple Cider Vinegar)

1/4 cup vinegar

1. After washing hair as normal, for final rinse gently rub vinegar into scalp.

2. Try as a daily treatment, even if you do not wash hair. Just rub vinegar into scalp and air dry.

Hair: Dandruff
(Apple Cider Vinegar)

1/4 cup vinegar
1/4 cup water

1. After washing and rinsing hair as usual, give hair a second rinse made of vinegar and water.

2. •Do not rinse this final solution out.

Hair: Dandruff Deep Treatment
(Apple Cider Vinegar)

1 cup vinegar, divided
2 pulverized aspirin
1 quart warm water

1. Combine 1/2 cup vinegar and aspirin.

2. Wash and rinse hair as usual.

3. Comb solution through hair and allow to condition hair follicles for 5 minutes before rinsing clean.

4. Add second 1/2 cup of vinegar to warm water and use as a final rinse for hair.

Hair Frizzy and Dry
(Apple Cider Vinegar)

1/2 cup vinegar
1 cup warm water

1. Combine vinegar and warm water together in a cup.

2. Shampoo hair as normal; use conditioner if necessary.

3. For final rinse, pour warm vinegar solution over hair and scalp.

Hair Moisturizer
(Apple Cider Vinegar)

1/2 cup vinegar, divided
2 teaspoon honey
1 egg yolk
1/3 cup olive oil

1. Combine all ingredients (using only 1/4 cup of the vinegar) and mix together until well incorporated.

2. Gently rub mixture into hair and scalp prior to washing.

3. Wrap treated hair in a wet towel.

4. Allow to set in hair for 10 minutes.

5. Shampoo as usual.

6. Rinse in lukewarm water with 1/4 cup of additional vinegar added.

Hair: Maintain Richness
(Apple Cider Vinegar)

4 teaspoons vinegar
4 teaspoons black strap molasses
4 teaspoons honey
8 ounces water

1. Combine all ingredients into a tall drinking glass.

2. Begin each day by drinking this concoction to maintain rich, healthy hair.

Hair Hot Oil Treatment
(Apple Cider Vinegar)

1/2 cup vinegar
1/4 cup olive oil
hot water

1. Heat olive oil until warm; massage into hair allowing more oil on ends and hair strands, and less into scalp.

2. Fill a bathroom sink or bowl with hot tap water.

3. Add vinegar to tub of water.

4. Soak a bath towel in vinegar water and wring it out by hand.

5. Wrap the wet, warm towel around hair.

6. Allow to soak for 20 – 30 minutes.

7. Remove towel and wash hair as normal.

8. Great treatment to repeat as part of your monthly beauty regimen (more often for particularly dry or damaged hair).

Hair: After Bath Rinse
(Apple Cider Vinegar)

1/2 cup vinegar
1/4 cup water

1. Following a shower or bath, give hair a final rinse with vinegar and water mixture; do not re-rinse but allow to dry.

Hair: Hair loss
(Apple Cider Vinegar)

1 teaspoon vinegar
6 ounces water

1. Combine vinegar and water.

2. Consume this mixture once a day, for 4 to 6 weeks; new hair follicles should begin to appear.

Radiant Skin
(Apple Cider Vinegar)

1/4 cup vinegar
3 large strawberries

1. Mash strawberries into vinegar and let sit undisturbed for two hours.

2. Strain strawberry-vinegar solution through a cloth and discard lumps.

3. Before bed, pat strawberry flavored vinegar onto face and neck.

4. In the morning, wash solution off face with normal cleansing routine.

Facial
(Apple Cider Vinegar)

1 cup vinegar
clean towel

1. Heat vinegar and bring to a boil.

2. Remove vinegar from stove and carefully pour hot vinegar into a large bowl.

3. Lean over the bowl, draping a towel over your head and the bowl.

4. Allow the warm steam to soften facial skin; remain with face over bowl until steaming action has ended.

5. After vinegar has cooled and you are no longer able to use it for steaming, dab a little of the vinegar onto face as a cleaning astringent.

Facial
(Apple Cider Vinegar)

1/2 cup vinegar
1/4 cup oatmeal
1/4 cup cooked rice

1. Combine all ingredients in a medium bowl until thoroughly combined.

2. Pat mixture onto face and neck.

3. Allow to dry, about 10 minutes.

4. Wash off paste with lukewarm water.

5. Rinse with cool water and gently pat skin dry with a clean, soft towel.

Facial
(Apple Cider Vinegar)

1 tablespoon vinegar
1 tablespoon honey
1/2 mashed banana
1/2 mashed peach

1. Mix ingredients until a sticky paste forms.

2. Apply coating to face and neck.

3. Allow to dry, about 10 minutes.

4. Rinse clean and pat dry.

Moisturizing Facial Mask
(Apple Cider Vinegar)

1 tablespoon vinegar
1 tablespoon honey
1/4 cup oatmeal

1. Combine ingredients until well mixed.

2. Gently pat mixture onto wet facial skin.

3. Allow to air dry.

4. Rinse off with cool water; apply moisturizer.

Facial Toner
(Apple Cider Vinegar)

1/2 cup vinegar
1/2 cup water

1. Combine vinegar and water in a plastic bottle.

2. Use cotton ball to apply to face daily.

Skin Protection
(Apple Cider Vinegar)

2 teaspoons vinegar
2 teaspoons olive oil

1. Combine vinegar and olive oil.

2. Gently pat onto clean facial skin before going outdoors to help protect from sun drying.

Skin: Itchy, Dry Skin
(Apple Cider Vinegar)

3 cups vinegar
bath full of warm water
handful of fresh thyme (optional)

1. Fill bathtub full of warm water and add vinegar.

2. Sprinkle handful of thyme over the water.

3. Soak in vinegar bath once a day to relieve all-over dry, itchy skin.

Skin: Lightening
(White Vinegar)

1/4 cup vinegar
1/4 cup lemon juice
1/2 cup white wine
1 tablespoon honey

1. Combine all ingredients and mix until well incorporated; store in jar or bottle.

2. Gently apply to face twice a day by blotting vinegar with a cotton ball.

Skin: Age (Liver) Spots
(Apple Cider Vinegar)

2 teaspoons vinegar
1 teaspoon onion juice

1. Combine ingredients together.

2. Apply directly to age spots daily.

3. Age spots should begin to fade in a few weeks.

Skin: Wrinkles
(Apple Cider Vinegar)

1 cup vinegar
1 tablespoon fennel seeds

1. Combine vinegar and fennel seeds, and heat over medium heat until hot.

2. Allow to simmer for 30 minutes, uncovered; some of the moisture will evaporate out.

3. Remove from heat and allow to cool completely.

4. Pour into a jar with a tight fitting lid.

5. Saturate a cotton ball with fennel-infused vinegar and gently dabbing over face and neck.

6. For even greater soothing action, gently heat jar of fennel vinegar in microwave before using.

7. Use warm vinegar and fennel combination to dab over wrinkles, allow for greater moisturizing penetration.

8. Use once or twice a day.

Skin: Age (Liver) Spots
(Apple Cider Vinegar)

1 tablespoon vinegar
1/2 onion

1. Dab cut side of onion into vinegar.

2. Gently rub directly onto age spots once a day.

3. Age spots should begin fading in a few weeks.

Skin: Pimples
(Apple Cider Vinegar)

1 teaspoon vinegar
1 teaspoon honey
1 tablespoon cornstarch

1. Combine all ingredients and blend together to form a thick paste.

2. Use paste on pimples and blackheads by gently rubbing (in a circular motion) on blemishes.

Skin: Herbal Bath Soak
(Apple Cider Vinegar)

Add chamomile to a vinegar bath, or substitute your favorite herbal vinegar such as peppermint or ginger.

3/4 cup vinegar
3 tablespoons chamomile

1. Add vinegar and chamomile to warm bath water.

2. Enjoy relaxing soak for at least 20 minutes.

Skin: Soothing Bath
(Apple Cider Vinegar)

1/4 cup vinegar
2 tablespoons favorite shampoo
1 cup olive oil

1. Combine all ingredients together and store in a plastic bottle.

2. Add 1/4 cup mixture to warm bath water for a soothing bath.

3. For variation, replace apple cider vinegar with tonics such as lavender or woodruff herbal vinegar.

After-Shower Body Wash to Balance pH
(Apple Cider Vinegar)

1/2 cup vinegar
1/2 cup water

1. Combine both ingredients together.

2. Use to rub down your body after bathing; solution will leave your skin silky soft as it balances pH levels, and free from drying soap film.

Skin: Balancing pH Levels
(Apple Cider Vinegar)

2 teaspoons vinegar
clean cloth or towelette

1. Soak clean cloth or towelette in vinegar.

2. Gently apply to face daily to balance pH levels.

Skin: Softening Skin Bath
(Apple Cider Vinegar)

1 cup vinegar
2 herbal tea bags
bath water

1. Simmer tea bags in vinegar on stove for 10 minutes.

2. Add to bath for soothing, softening skin bath.

Body Deodorizer
(Apple Cider Vinegar)

1/4 cup vinegar
1/2 cup water

1. Combine both ingredients in a cup or small bowl.

2. After shower or bath, use to rub down high odor areas of your body, such as under arms.

Skin: After Shave for Men
(White Vinegar)

Great herbs are thyme, sage, bay leaves, or cloves. Also add bee balm, chamomile and spearmint.

1 cup vinegar
2 tablespoons honey
1 tablespoon favorite herb

1. Mix ingredients in a small jar and seal with lid.

2. Allow to set for up to one week.

3. Strain out floating herbs.

4. Daily aftershave is now ready to use.

Skin: Men's Skin Bracer
(White Vinegar)

2 tablespoons vinegar
1/2 teaspoon cream of tartar
1/3 cup warm water

1. Combine all ingredients together.

2. Wash face, pat dry.

3. Gently pat bracer onto skin.

Skin: Cooling After Shave for Men
(White Vinegar)

1 cup vinegar
2 tablespoons honey
1 small cucumber
mint leaves

1. Place cucumber with peel in a blender along with fresh mint leaves.

2. Puree to a fine mixture.

3. Combine all ingredients, including cucumber, in a small jar and seal with lid.

4. Place in refrigerator overnight.

5. Strain out any cucumber peel or floating herbs using a sieve.

6. Pour tonic into a glass or plastic decanter, preferably one using a pump action dispenser; daily aftershave is now ready to use.

7. Keep refrigerated until use.

Hand Softener
(Apple Cider Vinegar)

1 tablespoon vinegar
2 cups warm water
1/2 teaspoon petroleum jelly

1. Add vinegar to warm water.

2. Soak hands in bowl for 5 minutes

3. Pat dry with a soft cloth.

4. Smooth petroleum jelly over hands and cover with clean cotton gloves.

5. Wear overnight; by morning hands will be unbelievably soft and smooth.

Hand Softener
(Apple Cider Vinegar)

1 teaspoon vinegar
1/2 cup water
1/2 teaspoon white sugar
1 teaspoon baby oil

1. Crudely combine all ingredients and then pour over hands.

2. Work this mixture into hands for 2 minutes, covering all parts of hands including backs, palms and between fingers.

3. Wash with a mild soap.

4. Use daily or as needed.

Soiled Hands
(Either Type)

1 tablespoon vinegar
1 teaspoon cornmeal

1. Wet soiled hands with vinegar.

2. Sprinkle cornmeal into both hands and rub vigorously together.

3. Rinse in cool water and pat dry.

Nail Trimming
(Apple Cider Vinegar)

Try this to soften nails immediately prior to trimming.

3 tablespoons vinegar
4 cups warm water

1. Combine vinegar and warm water.

2. Soak feet and toes in solution for 10 minutes.

3. Dry feet and proceed to trimming toe nails.

Nails: Beautiful Polish
(White Vinegar)

Your favorite nail polish will go on smoother and stay on days longer with this quick vinegar trick.

1 teaspoon vinegar
cotton ball

1. Clean uncoated fingernails with vinegar and allow to air dry.

2. Paint with favorite polish.

Rectal Itching
(Apple Cider Vinegar)

1/8 cup vinegar
thick gauze square

1. Soak clean gauze in vinegar.

2. Apply vinegar gauze directly to itch for relief.

3. Repeat as often as needed.

Armpit Odor
(Apple Cider Vinegar)

2-3 tablespoons of vinegar
clean cloth or paper towel

1. Soak cloth or paper towel in undiluted vinegar.

2. Clean armpits with vinegar cloth, but do not rinse; allow to air dry.

Foot Odor
(Apple Cider Vinegar)

1 cup apple cider vinegar
1 cup warm water

1 quart strong, warm tea

1. Soak feet in a pan of strong, warm tea for about 5 minutes.

2. Remove feet and rinse with warm water and vinegar.

3. Pat dry.

Foot Odor
(Apple Cider Vinegar)

1/4 cup vinegar
cotton balls or clean cloth

1. Wipe down feet twice daily with undiluted vinegar.

2. Do not dry, but allow to air dry.

Foot Softener
(Apple Cider Vinegar)

1/2 cup vinegar
bucket of warm water
favorite body lotion

1. Add vinegar to bucket of warm water.

2. Soak feet for 10 – 15 minutes; pat dry.

3. Apply favorite body lotion to feet and cover with clean pair of cotton socks.

Corns and Calluses
(Apple Cider Vinegar)

1/8 cup vinegar
stale bread
cotton ball

1. Soak bread with vinegar until mushy.

2. Apply vinegar-bread paste to cotton ball.

3. Secure in place over corn or callus and allow to remain overnight.

4. Repeat until corn or callus disappears.

Corns and Calluses
(Apple Cider Vinegar)

1/2 cup vinegar
bucket of warm water
1 tablespoon white sugar
baby oil
mild soap

1. Add vinegar to bucket of warm water.

2. Soak feet for 5 minutes.

3. Remove feet from bucket and, while still wet, rub white sugar onto bottoms of feet and any area bothered by corns or calluses; massage gently into skin.

4. Add a bit of baby oil and continue rubbing into feet.

5. Wash feet with a mild soap and cover with cotton socks.

Warts
(Apple Cider Vinegar)

1 teaspoon vinegar
small cotton gauze or cotton ball
tape

1. Soak piece of cotton gauze or cotton ball in vinegar.

2. Place soaked cotton ball on wart and tape into place.

3. Leave on wart for 30 minutes, twice a day until wart is gone.

Sunburns
(Apple Cider Vinegar)

1 cup vinegar
lukewarm bathtub of water

1. Fill bathtub with lukewarm water, taking care to not allow temperature to get too hot.

2. Add vinegar.

3. Soak 15-20 minutes for relief of sunburn pain.

Sunburns
(Apple Cider Vinegar)

vinegar, undiluted
clean cloth

1. Saturate a clean cloth with vinegar.

2. Gently place on sunburned skin for relief.

Mouthwash
(Either Type)

Apple cider vinegar can be used for any healing that needs to take place in the mouth; white vinegar can be used tor more intense flavor.

2 tablespoons vinegar
1/8 teaspoon peppermint flavoring (not oil)
8 ounces warm water

1. Add vinegar and peppermint flavoring to glass of warm water.

2. Gargle and rinse mouth clean.

Denture Cleaner
(Either Type)

White vinegar can be used in this formula, or apple cider vinegar for a refreshing twist.

1/2 teaspoon vinegar
6 ounces of water

1. Combine vinegar and water.

2. Allow dentures to soak overnight.

Denture Cleaner
(White Vinegar)

Using vinegar as a brush-on denture cleaner will not only remove lingering odors, but also help brighten dentures.

1 teaspoon vinegar

1. Brush dentures thoroughly using vinegar.

2. Rinse and air dry.

Weight Loss
(Apple Cider Vinegar)

2 teaspoons vinegar
8 ounce glass of water

1. Stir vinegar into glass of water.

2. Drink full glass of vinegar water 20 minutes before mealtime to suppress appetite and stimulate weight loss.

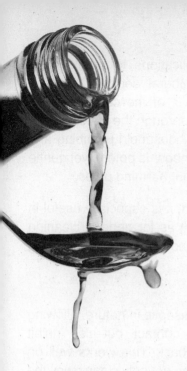

Chapter Six

Vinegar Around The Home

One of the greatest qualities vinegar possesses has long been its amazing ability to clean and disinfect. Hospitals, schools, nursing homes and day care centers have depended on vinegar to keep the standard of cleaning up, while bringing the occurrence of bacterial spread down. The results have been legendary.

But how does vinegar actually work as a household cleaner, and how can we use vinegar to its fullest potential?

Many of the same properties that make vinegar an excellent source of natural healing also contribute to making vinegar a workhorse of a cleaning agent. Vinegar's composition is a potent, non-poisonous liquid which is perfect for breaking down calcium carbonate and other mineral deposits. Its use is multi-purpose, making it the go-to product for a gamut of endeavors.

For example, vinegar not only pulls calcium from bones in cooking recipes to make a fortified broth (see the recipe for chicken soup in the cooking section of this book), but that same quality is harnessed in cleaning applications to break down calcium carbonate. This, and other mineral deposits, are the natural occurrence found in many areas of the country where "hard water" carries limestone particles through the water supply. These microscopic particles adhere to household plumbing and drains and eventually cause build up. Vinegar is potent, yet gentle enough, to remove these deposits without harming pipes.

Because vinegar itself is acid-based, it is especially useful in removing many types of stains, as well as for general cleaning applications such as washing dishes and glassware or cleaning glass to a streak-free shine.

Antibacterial and Antiseptic

Vinegar is both antibacterial and antiseptic in nature, allowing it to not only kill harmful bacteria on contact, but also inhibit bacteria's ability to successfully grow back. This works well on mold and mildew, where it is imperative to not only clean away the harmful fungus, but also destroy it at its root source.

Once an area is disinfected and cleaned with vinegar, germs have a difficult time regrouping on the same item. Not only is it clean to the naked eye, but the underlying bacteria has also been killed and removed.

Which Vinegar Works Best?

In most cleaning applications, white or distilled vinegar is the product of choice. For the sake of simplicity, we will be referring to the white vinegar name in this book. Truly, any vinegar will do the job for cleaning, but due to the greater volume used, white vinegar is much less expensive for cleaning purposes.

Vinegar in the Place of Chemical Cleaning Products

Cleaning with vinegar is especially useful for those people struggling with asthma or allergic conditions, as well as those with a sensitivity to certain chemical products.

Commercial cleaners contain a host of chemicals which can be harmful to the body or toxic when combined with other cleaning products. These products can leave residue behind, meaning that even though the area appears to be clean, toxins could linger long after using, exposing you and your family to potentially dangerous chemicals. Some scientists have wondered if the chemicals themselves are more dangerous than the bacteria they were designed to eliminate. Vinegar is all natural. Not only is it a chemical-free choice for home cleaning, it is safe for the environment and biodegradable, keeping our streams and riverbeds clean.

It is also safe for use around children and pets. After all, vinegar can be eaten! How many chemical cleaners can boast that fact?

How to Get Started

In using the formulas in this chapter, you may wish to get a head start by gathering a few common household items:

- Plastic spray bottle (2 cup version)
- Small fine mist sprayer (empty, trial size pump sprays work great for this)
- Discarded toothbrush
- Cotton swabs
- Soft cleaning rags, towels and/or sponges
- Nylon scrubbers
- Scrub brush

A Word About Vinegar Safety

Like all good things, vinegar does have its limitations. While vinegar is an amazing choice for cleaning virtually anything, there are a few instances when vinegar should not be used:

- Silver
- Pearls
- Blood stains
- Milk
- Vomit
- Butter
- Eggs
- Grease (vinegar is an excellent option for cutting grease, but not removing a grease STAIN)

As with anything you are using for the first time, always test these formulas in an inconspicuous area for sensitivity.

And, while vinegar is excellent for cleaning tarnished copper, great care should be taken to properly dispose of cleaning rags containing the buffed out green tarnish, as it is poisonous.

While vinegar is considered highly safe, there is always the chance that someone may develop a sensitivity to its contact. If you feel there is a chance that you may be allergic to vinegar, stop its use immediately and speak with your healthcare provider.

Grab a bucket, and let's get started!

Laundry: Pretreater
(White Vinegar)

This is a great pretreater for laundry stains. However, this pretreater should not be stored indefinitely in the spray bottle, as the ingredients may damage the pump spray.

4 tablespoons vinegar
3 tablespoons ammonia
2 tablespoons baking soda
1 tablespoon liquid detergent
cool water
spray bottle

1. Pour vinegar, ammonia and liquid detergent in spray bottle.

2. Mix together by gently shaking.

3. Add baking soda.

4. When reaction stops foaming, add water.

5. Use immediately to spray as a pretreater.

Laundry: Remove Clothing Manufacturing Chemicals
(White Vinegar)

1/4 cup vinegar
wash load

1. Add vinegar to laundry's wash cycle when washing new clothes for the first time; this will help eliminate any chemical residue from the manufacturing process.

2. Run through rinse cycle as usual.

Laundry: Clean and Whiten
(White Vinegar)

1/2 cup vinegar
wash load

1. Add undiluted vinegar to laundry's wash cycle to clean and whiten clothes; adding vinegar will also help kill any fungus growth and inhibit mold.

2. Run through rinse cycle as usual.

Laundry: Angora
(White Vinegar)

2 tablespoons vinegar
sink basin with clean, cool water

1. After washing, rinse angora in basin of clean water with vinegar added.

2. Gently remove excess water, without wringing, and lay flat to dry.

Laundry: Wool Sweaters
(White Vinegar)

1 cup vinegar

1. Add vinegar to laundry machine's rinse cycle.

2. Run as normal; wool sweaters will come out fluffier after vinegar rinse.

Laundry: Cotton
(White Vinegar)

3/4 cup vinegar

1. Add vinegar to laundry machine's rinse cycle.

2. Run as normal for softer cotton clothing; great for cotton blankets and sheets, too.

Laundry: Silks
(White Vinegar)

2 tablespoons vinegar

1. Add vinegar to final rinse cycle.

2. Do not rinse vinegar out.

Laundry: Alpaca Fabric
(White Vinegar)

1 tablespoon vinegar
tub or basin of water

1. After washing, rinse alpaca fabric in water to which vinegar has been added.

Laundry: Angora
(White Vinegar)

2 tablespoons vinegar
sink basin with clean, cool water

1. After washing, rinse angora in basin of clean water with vinegar added.

2. Gently remove excess water and lay flat to dry.

Laundry: Gentle Stain Removal
(White Vinegar)

3 tablespoons vinegar
3 tablespoons milk

1. Combine ingredients together in a small bowl.

2. Pour onto stain and gently rub fabric together.

3. Allow to sit for 5 minutes.

4. Wash as usual.

Laundry: Ink Stain Removal
(White Vinegar)

1 tablespoon vinegar
1 tablespoon cornstarch
milk; enough to cover stain

1. Soak ink stain in milk for one hour.

2. Combine vinegar and cornstarch into a paste.

3. Cover the stain with paste and rub into cloth.

4. Leave stain until the paste dries; wash normally.

Laundry: Permanent Press Stains
(White Vinegar)

vinegar, undiluted

1. Thoroughly wet stain with vinegar.

2. Allow to set for 3 – 5 minutes.

3. Wash in cool water and rinse clean.

Laundry: Perspiration Stains
(White Vinegar)

1/4 cup vinegar
2 gallons water

1. Combine vinegar and water in a clean sink.

2. Soak perspiration stained clothing in solution overnight.

3. Wash as usual.

Laundry: Wet Coffee and Tea Stains
(White Vinegar)

vinegar, undiluted
clean water
liquid detergent

1. Blot out as much coffee or tea as possible with a paper towel.

2. Rinse in cool water.

3. Pour vinegar directly onto stain.

4. Wash in lukewarm, soapy water.

Laundry: Dry Coffee and Tea Stains
(White Vinegar)

vinegar, undiluted

1. Soak stain in undiluted vinegar for 30 minutes.

2. Wash as normal to finish removing stain.

3. If stain has not come out, repeat process again before drying.

Laundry: Dark Coffee and Tea Stains
(White Vinegar)

vinegar, undiluted
1 teaspoon salt

1. Wet stained area with vinegar.

2. Sprinkle dampened stain with salt.

3. Set stained garment in bright sunlight for at least one hour.

4. Wash and dry clothing as usual.

5. For toughest stains, you may need to repeat this process.

Laundry: Wine Stains
(White Vinegar)

vinegar, undiluted

1. Blot undiluted vinegar on a wine stain; stain will begin to dissipate and fade away.

2. Wash as usual.

Laundry: Red Wine Stains
(White Vinegar)

This is a good formula for removing the tough wine stains. Be careful to work gently with delicate fabrics.

1 tablespoon vinegar
3 tablespoons water
1 teaspoon salt

1. Blot up as much wine as possible from fabric.

2. Saturate stain with vinegar and water.

3. While stain is wet with vinegar solution, gently rub salt into stain.

4. Set in sunlight to dry.

5. Wash as normal.

Laundry: Iron Scorching Stains
(White Vinegar)

vinegar, undiluted
1 teaspoon salt
clean cloth

1. Dampen a clean cloth with undiluted vinegar.

2. Blot vinegar onto scorched area and allow to set for 5 minutes.

3. Repeat if scorching remains.

4. If after 2 attempts, scorching still remains, sprinkle salt over remoistened scorch and allow to set for 5 minutes.

5. Wash as normal.

Laundry: Rust Stains
(White Vinegar)

1 tablespoon vinegar
1 teaspoon salt

1. Pour vinegar over rust stain, using enough vinegar to cover stain entirely.

2. Sprinkle salt over dampened stain.

3. Set outside in the sun for at least an hour to dry.

4. Rinse out salt and reapply until stain disappears completely.

5. Wash as usual.

Laundry: Musty Smell from Bedding or Drapes
(Apple Cider Vinegar)

Vinegar, undiluted
soft cloth or hand towel

1. Saturate cloth or hand towel with vinegar, and wring out.

2. Place musty bedding in clothes dryer along with vinegared cloth.

3. Set clothes dryer setting to "Air Dry" and run for 5 – 10 minutes, allowing vinegared cloth to soak up musty odors.

4. Repeat, if necessary, or hang outside to complete drying.

Laundry: Deodorize Cigarette or Cigar Smoke
(White Vinegar)

2 cups vinegar
Tub of very hot water

1. After washing clothing, hang odored clothing above tub.

2. Pour vinegar into tub of very hot water.

3. Allow steam to rid clothing of smoke.

4. Repeat if necessary.

Laundry: Eliminate Static Cling
(White Vinegar)

1/4 cup vinegar
rinse load

1. Add vinegar to the laundry's rinse cycle to eliminate static cling and reduce lint.

Laundry: Setting Fabric Dyes
(White Vinegar)
Use this formula to "set" dye after coloring

1 cup white vinegar
1 gallon cold water
1 teaspoon salt

1. Fill bucket or sink with cold water, vinegar and salt.

2. Soak newly dyed fabric in solution for 1 hour.

3. Rinse in cold water to set dye.

Laundry: Natural Red Dye Coloring
(White Vinegar)

This formula allows you to make your very own natural red dye for fabrics.

1/2 cup vinegar
1 pound beets
1 quart water

1. Wash beets and place them in a saucepan, and cover with cool water.

2. Simmer until beets are tender; remove skins.

3. Chop beets and return to same water in which they were cooked.

4. Allow beets to set in water for 2 hours.

5. Strain off red liquid and combine with vinegar to achieve a natural red dye.

Laundry: Diapers
(White Vinegar)

This is a good formula for use in washing baby's cloth diapers. Vinegar will help discourage diaper rashes on baby's bottom.

3/4 cup vinegar

1. Add vinegar to final rinse water for diapers (diapers should always be rinsed twice)

2. No not add fabric softeners to baby's diaper rinse, as chemicals softeners may irritate baby's delicate skin. Softeners also make diapers less absorbing.

Laundry: Easy Rinse
(White Vinegar)

These presoaked cloths are easy to add to the final rinse cycle. They not only save measuring each time, but keep vinegar from directly contacting delicate fabrics.

vinegar, undiluted
clean washcloths
plastic container with lid or sealing plastic bag

1. Soak washcloths in vinegar until saturated.

2. Place cloths, one on top of another, in small plastic container or zipping plastic baggie.

3. Toss in one of these preloaded cloths into final rinse cycle of your washing machine.

Laundry: Fabric Softener, Scent-Free
(White Vinegar)

1/3 cup vinegar
1/3 cup baking soda

1. Combine vinegar and baking soda in a cup.

2. Add to final rinse water for soft, scent-free laundry.

Laundry: Fabric Softener, Scented
(Apple Cider Vinegar)

1/2 cup vinegar
1/3 cup baking soda

1. Combine vinegar and baking soda in a cup.

2. Add to final rinse water for a scented softener.

Laundry: Fabric Softener, Gentle
(White Vinegar)

Use this for scent-free laundry. Excellent for people who are allergic to chemical softeners.

1/3 cup vinegar

1. Add vinegar to final rinse cycle.

Laundry: Straw Hats
(White Vinegar)

Straw hats can become worn out and misshapen. Try this formula to bring new life to old straw hats.

1 teaspoon vinegar
1/2 cup salt
bucket of water plus 1 cup water
few drops liquid detergent, if necessary
spray bottle

1. Put salt in bucket of warm water and dissolve.

2. Submerge straw hat in salt water.

3. Once straw is slightly softened, remove from salt water and wipe away stains.

4. For tough stains, add a drop or two of liquid detergent to a sponge and wipe clean.

5. Push and mold hat back into original shape.

6. Put vinegar and 1 cup water in a spray bottle.

7. Once hat is in desired shape, spray hat with a fine mist of vinegar solution.

8. Allow to air dry, but do not dry in direct sunlight.

Laundry: Panty Hose Revitalizer
(White Vinegar)

This formula works wonders on stretched out panty hose.

1/4 cup vinegar
1 quart warm water

1. In a small bowl or clean sink basin, combine vinegar and warm water.

2. Soak panty hose for 5 minutes.

3. Remove and gently squeeze out excess moisture (do not wring).

4. Blot with a towel.

5. Allow panty hose to dry, spread out flat on a towel to help soak up water.

Laundry: Lint Trap
(White Vinegar)

Hard water can cause mineral buildup on washing machine lint traps. Use this formula to occasionally clean the trap.

Vinegar, undiluted
cleaning brush

1. Soak lint trap in undiluted vinegar for 2 hours.

2. Brush mineral deposits clean with a cleaning brush.

3. Rinse and replace.

Laundry: Saddle Soap
(White Vinegar)

1/4 cup vinegar
1/8 cup liquid soap
1/8 cup linseed oil
1/4 cup beeswax

1. Warm the beeswax slowly, over medium heat, and add vinegar.

2. Add soap and oil, and stir together.

3. Keep the mixture warm until it all blends into a smooth mixture.

4. Remove from heat and cool on countertop until it reaches a solid state.

5. When ready to use, rub saddle soap into leather; then buff to a high shine with a soft, clean cloth.

Laundry: Polish Leather
(White Vinegar)

1/3 cup vinegar
2/3 cup linseed oil
1/3 cup water
2 soft cloths

1. Combine all ingredients together in a bowl or small tub.

2. Apply to leather with a soft cloth.

3. Using a second, clean cloth, buff to a high shine.

Laundry: Leather Cleaning
(White Vinegar)

1/2 cup vinegar
2-3 vitamin E capsules
1/2 cup olive oil

1. Bring vinegar to a boil.

2. Add vitamin capsules allowing to dissolve.

3. Add olive oil and blend all ingredients.

4. Use to clean leather coats.

Laundry: Leather Shoes
(White Vinegar)

1 tablespoon vinegar
1 tablespoon rubbing alcohol
1 teaspoon vegetable oil
3-4 drops liquid soap

1. Combine all ingredients.

2. Wipe solution onto leather shoes; buff until clean.

Laundry: Patent Leather Shoes
(White Vinegar)

vinegar, undiluted
1 teaspoon petroleum jelly
paper towel

1. Moisten a paper towel with undiluted vinegar.

2. Gently rub into clean patent leather shoes.

3. Finish by rubbing a slight amount of petroleum jelly into leather and buff to a beautiful shine.

Laundry: Saddles and Boots
(White Vinegar)

1/4 cup vinegar
beeswax, enough to make into a cleaning paste
few drops of liquid soap
few drops of oil

1. Work beeswax into warm vinegar.

2. Add soap and oil.

3. Heat until all ingredients are soft and mixed together; cool completely.

4. Use to clean horse saddles and cowboy boots.

Laundry: Removing/Adding Hems to Clothing
(White Vinegar)

vinegar, undiluted
iron

1. Dampen letdown hems with vinegar prior to ironing to eliminate creases.

2. To add creases to fabric or hems, again dampen with vinegar and iron in a new crease.

Kitchen: Cutting Boards
(White Vinegar)

2 tablespoons vinegar
paper towel

1. Wipe down cutting boards with undiluted vinegar.

2. Allow to air dry.

Kitchen: Cutting Board and Cutting Blocks
(White Vinegar)

vinegar, undiluted
1 tablespoon baking soda
spray bottle

1. Sprinkle baking soda over wooden cutting board or block and rub into wood.

2. Spray baking soda with undiluted vinegar.

3. Let stand for 5 minutes.

4. Rinse with clean water, allowing solution to bubble.

5. Rinse away and dry.

Kitchen: Cutting Board Deep Sanitization
(White Vinegar)

1/2 cup vinegar
2-3 tablespoons salt
2 teaspoons vegetable oil (for wood cutting boards)

1. Apply salt to coat cutting board (using more if necessary) and allow to set for 5-10 minutes

2. Scrub salt with a vinegar wash.

3. Rinse well using hot water.

4. Dry with a cloth.

5. For wood cutting boards, occasionally rub in vegetable oil to keep wood like new.

Kitchen: Counter Disinfectant
(White Vinegar)

3 tablespoons vinegar
1 teaspoon liquid soap
1/2 teaspoon oil
1/2 cup water

1. Combine all ingredients.

2. Using a wash towel, wipe down kitchen counters to thoroughly disinfect.

Kitchen: Countertops
(White Vinegar)

vinegar, undiluted
paper towels

1. Soak a paper towel in undiluted vinegar.

2. Lay the soaked towel on the caked area and allow to set for 30-60 minutes and wipe clean.

Kitchen: Countertops
(White Vinegar)

Make a bottleful of this natural cleaner to keep on hand every time you want to clean.

1 cup vinegar
1 cup water
spray bottle

1. Combine vinegar and water and store in a spray bottle.

2. Use this solution to wipe down kitchen countertops.

Kitchen: Countertops
(White Vinegar)

Keep this scrubber to keep on hand for easy clean up that will not damage countertop surface.

vinegar, undiluted
discarded nylon hosiery

1. Completely soak nylon hosiery in vinegar.

2. Use to scrub hard to clean areas of countertops.

Kitchen: Counter Stain Remover
(White Vinegar)

1/4 cup vinegar
1/4 cup water

1. Combine vinegar and water together and use to wipe down stained counter.

2. For difficult stains, allow cloth soaked in this solution to lay on top of stain for 15 minutes.

3. Then wipe clean.

Kitchen: Stainless Steel
(White Vinegar)

vinegar, undiluted
1 -2 tablespoons baking soda

1. Dampen a cleaning cloth with vinegar and dip into baking soda to coat.

2. Rub onto stainless steel in a circular motion.

3. Buff with dry side of cloth until shiny clean.

Kitchen: Stainless Steel
(White Vinegar)

vinegar, undiluted
soft cloth

1. Dampen soft cloth with undiluted vinegar.

2. Wipe down and clean stainless steel appliances.

3. Polish dry without rinsing.

Kitchen: Stainless Steel Sinks
(White Vinegar)

*Use this formula to clean rust stains from stainless
steel sink drains.*

1 tablespoon vinegar
1 teaspoon salt

1. Pour salt over rust stained spot in sink.

2. Drizzle vinegar over salt and clean with a paper
   towel or cleaning cloth.

Kitchen: Drains
(White Vinegar)

1/2 cup vinegar

1. Pour undiluted vinegar down each drain weekly
   to keep drains fresh and discourage clogging.

2. No need to rinse away.

Kitchen: Drains
(White Vinegar)

This is a great formula to freshen and open up slow moving drains.

1/2 cup vinegar
1/2 cup baking soda
hot water

1. Pour baking soda down drain.

2. Pour vinegar down drain on top of baking soda.

3. Allow to rest for 10 minutes.

4. Run hot water down drain to rinse clean.

Kitchen: Drains and Septics
(White Vinegar)

Use this formula once a month to keep drains running free and give a bacteria boost to septic systems.

drain cleaner formula (above)
1 package dry yeast
2/3 cup brown sugar

1. Using above formula for cleaning drains, treat each drain in the house.

2. After treating drains, proceed to treat septic tank.

3. Pour yeast and brown sugar into toilet and flush tank twice.

4. Doing this monthly will help keep the drain and septic system running efficiently for many years.

Kitchen: Garbage Disposal
(White Vinegar)

Clean and freshen garbage disposals with this weekly treatment.

1/2 cup vinegar
tray of ice cubes

1. Place tray of ice cubes in drain.

2. Pour vinegar over ice cubes.

3. Run water over cubes and vinegar while running garbage disposal.

Kitchen: Garbage Disposal
(Apple Cider Vinegar)

This formula is a twist to the garbage disposal formula above. "Disposal ice cubes" can be made in advance to keep for future use.

1/2 cup vinegar
1/2 cup water

1. Combine vinegar and water and fill ice cube tray; freeze.

2. Frozen vinegar cubes can be stored in a plastic zip bag in freezer for future use.

3. Grind a handful of these vinegar cubes each week to keep disposal blades sharp and disposal fresh.

Kitchen: Faucets and Fixtures
(White Vinegar)

1 tablespoon vinegar
1 tablespoons cream of tartar

1. Mix both ingredients into a paste.

2. Rub paste onto dingy faucets and kitchen fixtures and allow to dry completely.

3. Using a pan of warm, clean water, wash dried paste off fixtures and buff dry with a clean cloth.

Kitchen: Faucets and Fixtures
(White Vinegar)

1/3 cup vinegar
2/3 cup water

1. Combine vinegar and water.

2. Use soft cloth to polish and shine faucets and fixtures.

Kitchen: Appliances
(White Vinegar)

1/4 cup vinegar
1 teaspoon borax
2 cups hot water

1. Combine all ingredients and pour into a plastic spray bottle.

2. Spray vinegar solution on greasy smears on kitchen appliances.

3. Buff appliances in a circular motion with a soft cloth.

Kitchen: Black Appliances
(White Vinegar)

Black or dark colored appliances, like stainless steel, seem to show every fingerprint or smudge. They also tend to show swirl markings from cleaning. Try this formula to keep black appliances looking new and smudge free.

vinegar, undiluted
soft, lint-free cloth

1. Clean appliance as usual.

2. Using undiluted vinegar on a soft lint-free cloth, do a final wipe down of the appliance.

3. Buff with a clean cloth.

Kitchen: Microwave Ovens
(White Vinegar)

1/2 cup vinegar
1/2 cup water

1. In a small, microwave-safe bowl, heat vinegar and water in the microwave until it begins to boil.

2. Now run the microwave on its highest setting for 30 seconds.

3. Spills and baked on foods should now wipe down with ease.

4. For any additional cleaning, use a clean cloth and the rest of this vinegar solution (once it cools) to wipe away grime.

Kitchen: Microwave Oven Odor
(Apple Cider Vinegar)

3 tablespoons vinegar
1 cup water

1. Pour vinegar and water into a microwave-safe cup or bowl.

2. Bring vinegar mixture to a boil in the microwave.

3. Allow to set in closed microwave for 5 minutes.

4. Microwave will smell fresh and apple cider vinegar-clean.

Kitchen: Refrigerators
(White Vinegar)

Use this formula to remove any dirt or grease layer than has built up on the top of your refrigerator.

vinegar, undiluted
few drops liquid detergent
spray bottle

1. Spray undiluted vinegar on top of refrigerator and add a few drops of liquid detergent.

2. Using a cloth or sponge, give the entire appliance top a quick pat to make sure vinegar and detergent is in contact with any grease build up.

3. All to soak for 15 minutes.

4. Wipe clean with cloth or sponge.

5. Rinse with hot water and a tablespoon or two of additional vinegar and dry completely.

Kitchen: Refrigerator and Freezer Gaskets
(White Vinegar)

vinegar, undiluted
teaspoon liquid detergent
2 cups warm water

1. Squirt liquid detergent into water and use to wipe down refrigerator and freezer gaskets.

2. Use undiluted vinegar to wipe any mold clean.

3. Rinse and dry with a clean towel

Kitchen: Self-Defrosting Refrigerators
(White Vinegar)

1 tablespoon vinegar
few drops liquid detergent

1. Remove water collecting tray and wash in hot soapy water.

2. Dry tray and replace.

3. Add vinegar to water collecting tray to retard growth of bacteria and keep refrigerator fresh.

Kitchen: Gas Stove Grates
(White Vinegar)

1 cup vinegar
2 cups water

1. On a stove top, place individual iron grates from gas stove in a pot of vinegar and water.

2. Bring to a boil for 10 minutes.

3. Remove from vinegar water and wipe clean.

Kitchen: Stove Tops
(White Vinegar)

1/2 cup vinegar
1/2 cup water
1 teaspoon liquid detergent

1. Combine all ingredients together.

2. Using a soft cloth, wipe down stove tops to rid of cooked on food and grease.

3. Rinse clean with a cloth wet with water and buff dry.

Kitchen: Oven Racks
(White Vinegar)

1 cup vinegar, plus extra for spraying
1 tablespoon dish detergent
tub of hot water
spray bottle

1. Remove racks from oven and spray thoroughly with vinegar (you may wish to do this outdoors); allow racks to air dry.

2. Place racks in tub of very hot water, vinegar and dish detergent.

3. Allow racks to soak for 30 minutes; turn racks and repeat on opposite end if you are unable to fit entire rack in tub at one time.

4. You may need to soak racks a second time.

5. Wipe down racks with a cloth or sponge.

Kitchen: Oven Cleaner
(White Vinegar)

When using ammonia, you may wish to use rubber or plastic cleaning gloves to protect your hands.

1/2 cup white vinegar
3 cups water
2 cups ammonia
2 cups baking soda

1. Pour water in a shallow baking dish and place in oven.

2. Heat oven to 300°.

3. Turn off oven and allow water to remain in oven for 30 minutes.

4. After 30 minutes, remove baking dish and discard water.

5. Replace with ammonia, put back in warm oven (but turned off) and allow to set overnight.

6. In the morning, pour out all except 1/2 cup of ammonia.

7. Add vinegar and baking soda to remaining ammonia.

8. Use this mixture to wash down oven surfaces and then allow to set on oven surfaces for 30 minutes.

9. After 30 minutes, wipe away oven cleaner and rinse with clean water; dry.

Kitchen: Dishwashers
(White Vinegar)

When cleaning automatic dishwashers, be careful not to completely dry inside bottom of appliance. Some manufacturers depend on a small amount of remaining moisture to keep seals from drying out and cracking.

2 cups white vinegar
cleaning rag

1. Pour vinegar into bottom of empty dishwasher.

2. Run dishwasher without using any detergent, only the added vinegar.

3. When both wash and rinse cycles end, but before drying cycle begins, turn off appliance and wipe down the interior top, sides and dishwasher door with a cloth.

Kitchen: Exhaust Fan Grill
(White Vinegar)

vinegar, undiluted
clean cloth

1. Wash exhaust fan grill, removing any dust and debris.

2. Wet clean cloth with vinegar and wipe down fan grill to remove any remaining grease.

3. This will help retard future grease build up.

Small Appliances
(White Vinegar)

When cleaning small appliances, do not spray vinegar or any other liquid solution, directly onto the appliance. Moisture could enter the appliance's vent and damage internal parts. ALL appliances should be unplugged prior to cleaning.

vinegar, undiluted
clean cloths

1. Wipe down appliance with clean cloth saturated with white vinegar.

2. Use a second clean cloth to buff appliance dry.

Kitchen: Can Openers
(White Vinegar)

vinegar, undiluted
cotton swabs
bowl
soft cloth

1. Wipe down can opener with a soft cloth dipped in vinegar.

2. Soak removable opener blade in a small bowl of vinegar to remove encrusted food; carefully wipe clean.

3. Use a vinegar soaked cotton swab tip to clean can opener vents and operation buttons.

4. Wipe dry with a clean cloth.

Kitchen: Mixers
(White Vinegar)

Mixers seem to be one of the hardest kitchen appliances to keep clean. Try this handy formula for loosening dried on food.

vinegar, undiluted
soft cleaning cloth

1. Saturate clean cloth with vinegar.

2. Wrap vinegar soaked cloth around mixer and allow to set for 5 minutes.

3. Remove cloth and wipe clean.

Kitchen: Coffee Pots
(White Vinegar)

1 tablespoon vinegar
water

1. Fill coffee pot with water and add vinegar.

2. Allow to set for 10 minutes.

3. Rinse well.

Kitchen: Coffee Pots
(White Vinegar)

1 cup vinegar
1 cup water

1. Combine vinegar and water.

2. Run this combination through automatic coffee pot brewing cycle.

Kitchen: Coffee Pots
(White Vinegar)

1 tablespoon vinegar
2-3 drops dish detergent
water

1. In coffee receptacle, pour vinegar and detergent.

2. Run one pot of water through full brewing cycle.

3. Rinse pot several times with hot water.

Kitchen: Electric Knives
(White Vinegar)

vinegar, undiluted
few drops liquid detergent
soft cloth
toothpick

1. Wipe electric knife with a cloth dampened with vinegar and soapy water.

2. Saturate area around dirty blade mounting.

3. Use toothpick to scrape area clean.

4. Wipe electric cord and dry thoroughly.

Kitchen: Sharpen Knives
(White Vinegar)

vinegar, undiluted
spray bottle
clay pot

1. Spray vinegar onto the bottom of a clay pot.

2. Sharpen knife using clay pot as a whetstone.

Kitchen: Small Appliance Buttons
(White Vinegar)

Ever wonder how to clean small blender buttons and other appliance control knobs? Try this formula.

vinegar, undiluted
cottons swabs

1. Saturate tip of a cotton swab with vinegar.

2. Use to clean tops and around sides of small buttons and control knobs.

Kitchen: Appliance Cords
(White Vinegar)

vinegar, undiluted
soft cloths

1. Wet a soft cloth with vinegar.

2. Use to periodically wipe down appliance cords to keep free from food and other debris.

3. Dry with another soft cloth.

Kitchen: Clean Old Sponges
(White Vinegar)

1/4 cup vinegar
1 quart water

1. Rinse sponges in kitchen sink, and wring out.

2. Place water and vinegar in a bucket.

3. Put sponges in vinegar water and allow to soak clean overnight.

Kitchen: Deodorizer
(Apple Cider Vinegar)

vinegar, undiluted
clean cloth

1. Soak a clean cloth in apple cider vinegar and wring out any excess moisture.

2. Place wet cloth on top of heat or air register.

3. Allow air to circulate through moistened cloth for 30 minutes to make kitchen smell fresh and eliminate odors.

Kitchen: Deodorizer
(White Vinegar)

2 tablespoons vinegar
4 ounce pump bottle

1. Fill pump bottle with vinegar.

2. After cooking fish, cabbage or for boil overs, spray a few pumps of undiluted vinegar in the air to neutralize odor.

Kitchen: Eliminate Cooking Odors
(Either Type)

1/4 cup vinegar
1 teaspoon cinnamon (optional)

1. Simmer vinegar in an uncovered pot of water to clear the air of lingering cooking odors.

2. For a clean smell, use white vinegar.

3. For a special air freshened scent, use apple cider vinegar with cinnamon added.

Kitchen: Glassware
(White Vinegar)

1/4 cup vinegar
hot rinse water

1. Add vinegar to final rinse water.

2. After cleaning, soak glasses in hot vinegar water; remove and allow to air dry.

Dishes: Grease Cutter
(White Vinegar)

1/2 cup vinegar
warm to hot dishwater

1. Add vinegar to dishwater, using your favorite dish soap as usual.

2. Vinegar will work to cut heavy grease in the water for cleaner dishes.

Dishes: Copper and Brass Cleaner
(White Vinegar)

1/4 cup vinegar
1/4 cup lemon juice
paper towel
soft cloth

1. Combine both ingredients in a small bowl.

2. Apple mixture to copper or brass with a paper towel.

3. Buff to a beautiful shine with a soft cloth.

Dishes: Pewter
(White Vinegar)

1 tablespoon vinegar
1 tablespoon salt
1 tablespoon flour

1. Combine all three ingredients together, using just enough vinegar to form a paste.

2. Smear paste on discolored pewter and allow to dry completely.

3. Rub off the dried paste.

4. Rinse in hot water and buff completely dry.

Dishes: Pewter
(White Vinegar)

3 tablespoons vinegar
cabbage leaves
1 teaspoon salt

1. Soak cabbage leaves in vinegar.

2. Dip wet cabbage leaf in salt; use to buff pewter.

3. Rinse with cool water and dry pewter.

Dishes: Stuck on Food
(White Vinegar)

1/2 cup vinegar
1 1/2 cups water

1. Add vinegar water to pots with stuck on food.

2. Heat vinegar and water mixture in dirty pot, and wipe clean.

Dishes: Greasy Pots and Pans
(White Vinegar)

vinegar, undiluted
spray bottle

1. Place undiluted vinegar in a spray bottle.

2. Spray a thick coat of vinegar on greasy pans.

3. Allow to sit 3 – 5 minutes.

4. Grease will come off easier, using less dish soap.

Dishes: Aluminum Pots and Pans
(White Vinegar)

This formula is a great way to keep new aluminum pots and pans from discoloration.

1/2 cup vinegar
2 cups water

1. Pour vinegar and water into aluminum pan.

2. Bring to a boil.

3. Wipe pan clean.

Dishes: Aluminum Pots and Pans Stain
(White Vinegar)

1 tablespoon vinegar
1 teaspoon baking soda

1. Combine vinegar and baking soda into a paste.

2. Use this paste, cleaning in a circular motion, to remove light stains from cookware.

Dishes: Aluminum Pots and Pans Stain
(White Vinegar)

Try this for slightly heavier stains.

1 tablespoon vinegar
1 teaspoon baking soda
1 teaspoon cream of tartar

1. Combine all three ingredients and mix into a paste.

2. Rubbing in a circular motion, remove stains from cooking pots and pans.

Dishes: Aluminum Pots and Pans Stain
(White Vinegar)

This formula can be used for heavily stained aluminum.

1 tablespoon vinegar
1 tablespoon liquid detergent
1 teaspoon baking soda
1 teaspoon cream of tartar
nylon scrubbing pad

1. Combine all ingredients together and mix into a gritty gel.

2. Spread this gel over stains in pan and rub in a circular motion with nylon scrubbing pad to remove stains

3. Rinse well.

4. Repeat a second time, if necessary.

Dishes: Copper Pan Cleaner
(White Vinegar)

1 cup vinegar
1/2 cup powdered dish detergent
1/2 cup water
1/2 cup salt
1/4 cup flour

1. Combine all ingredients in a bowl, whisking until thoroughly blended.

2. Heat slowly in a double boiler until detergent is dissolved and mixture begins to thicken.

3. Remove from heat and cool completely.

4. Once cool, use this mixture to wipe onto a copper pot and coat.

5. Allow to set for 30 seconds.

6. Wipe clean with a soft cloth.

Dishes: Non Stick Pans
(White Vinegar)

Try this to remove mineral deposits and other stains from coated cookware without damaging the coating.

1/3 cup vinegar
2 cups water

1. Pour water and vinegar into non stick pan stained with mineral deposits.

2. Over medium heat, bring to a boil on stove top.

3. Allow to boil for at least 3 minutes.

4. Wipe pan clean with a soft cloth.

Dishes: Musty Glass Jars
(White Vinegar)

vinegar, undiluted
clean sponge

1. Dampen a clean sponge with vinegar and wring out any excess.

2. Place dampened sponge in jar and seal tightly with lid.

3. Leave to soak up musty odors for at least 30 minutes.

Dishes: Thermoses
(White Vinegar)

1 cup vinegar
1/2 cup water
1 tablespoon rice, uncooked

1. Fill thermos with water vinegar solution.

2. Fit with lid and shake to coat entire thermos bottle.

3. Let stand for 1 hour.

4. After hour, add rice and shake for an additional 2 minutes.

5. Pour out contents and rinse thoroughly.

6. Wipe dry.

Dishes: Stained Plastic Food Storage Containers
(White Vinegar)

1-2 tablespoons vinegar
1/4 cup water

1. Place vinegar in dirty or stained plastic food storage container.

2. Add water and use cloth to coat entire container.

3. Allow to sit 20 minutes.

4. Wipe clean and rinse.

Dishes: Plastic Food Storage Containers
(White Vinegar)

1/4 cup vinegar
1 teaspoon liquid detergent
1 quart warm water

1. Combine vinegar, detergent and warm water.

2. Use solution to soak plastic containers to rid them of food odors.

Dishes: Smelly Plastic Food Storage Containers
(White Vinegar)

2 tablespoons vinegar
paper towel

1. Moisten a paper towel with vinegar.

2. Place wet paper towel in storage container and seal shut with lid.

3. Allow to set overnight.

4. Remove paper towel and rinse.

Dishes: Automatic Dishwasher Rinse
(White Vinegar)

vinegar, undiluted

1. Pour undiluted vinegar in dishwasher's rinse cycle dispenser.

2. Run wash load as normal.

3. Refill rinse cycle with additional vinegar monthly, or as needed.

Dishes: Cloudy Drinkware
(White Vinegar)

vinegar, undiluted
small tub or wash basin
liquid dish detergent

1. Wash glasses and other drinkware as usual.

2. Fill a small tub or wash basin with undiluted vinegar.

3. Submerge glasses in vinegar tub and allow to soak for 30 minutes.

4. Remove from vinegar tub and gently wash with a scrub brush dipped in soapy water.

5. Rinse glasses in clean, hot water.

6. If necessary, rinse glasses a final time in a sink full of hot water to which 1/2 cup white vinegar has been added.

7. Dry with a soft cloth.

Dishes: Vases
(White Vinegar)

Flower vases can be difficult to clean due to their odd shape and narrow openings.

1/8 cup vinegar
nylon scrub brush

1. Pour vinegar into a small dish.

2. Use nylon scrub brush dipped in vinegar to clean hard to reach areas of vase interior.

3. Rinse with hot water.

Dishes: Vases
(White Vinegar)

This is an even better formula for the toughest to clean vases.

1/4 cup vinegar
1/4 cup hot water
3 tablespoons sand

1. Pour sand into vase opening.

2. Follow with vinegar and hot water.

3. Shake vase vigorously, removing dirt deposits from inside of vase.

4. Empty all contents from vase and rinse well before drying.

Dishes: Vases
(White Vinegar)

This is a great formula for vases with narrow openings that make it almost impossible to clean on the inside.

1/2 cup vinegar, plus 1/4 cup vinegar
1/4 cup uncooked rice
1/2 cup cold water
1/2 cup warm water

1. Pour rice into vase opening.

2. Follow rice with vinegar and cold water.

3. Shake vase, spinning it in a circular motion, then in reverse direction

4. Let set for 1 minute, and repeat shaking and spinning action.

5. Pour out rice and vinegar solution.

6. Rinse out vase with second half cup of vinegar and warm water.

7. Set upside down on counter to allow to dry.

Dishes: Ceramic Baking Dishes
(White Vinegar)

1/8 cup vinegar
nylon scrubber

1. Pour vinegar in a small bowl.

2. Use nylon scrubber to remove baked on food from ceramic bakeware.

3. Wash as usual.

Dishes: Enamel Baking Dishes
(White Vinegar)

2 cups vinegar

1. Wash all easy-to-remove food from enamel baking dish.

2. Pour in vinegar (if 2 cups is not enough to cover baked on food in dish, simply add a little more).

3. Place baking dish on stove top or in oven and bring vinegar to a boil in baking dish.

4. Boil for several minutes before removing from heat and allowing to cool.

5. Pour out vinegar and wash baking dish.

Dishes: Lead Crystal
(White Vinegar)

Lead crystal should always be washed by hand, not in the dishwasher.

1/4 cup vinegar
water
liquid detergent

1. Make a sink full of soapy water using warm to hot water and a few drops of liquid detergent.

2. Place a rubber tub mat in bottom of sink to keep lead crystal safe from chips and scratches.

3. Submerge lead crystal and wash thoroughly.

4. Rinse in sink full of hot water and vinegar.

5. If rinse water was hot, crystal will rapidly air dry on a clean towel or drying rack.

Dishes: Fine China
(White Vinegar)

Fine china should also be washed by hand. NOTE: This formula is for china that is free from gold or silver trim; vinegar is known to cause metal trim work to discolor.

1/4 cup vinegar
water
liquid detergent
paper plates or paper towels

1. Gently wash fine China by hand in warm soapy water.

2. Rinse in sink full of hot water and vinegar.

3. Dry each piece of China with a clean, soft cloth.

4. To store safely, place a paper plate or single paper towel between each piece of china to prevent chipping.

Floor Washing
(White Vinegar)

Vinegar can dissolve preexisting wax on floors. Use small amounts to achieve clean and shine; move to higher concentrations for wax and dirt build up.

2 cups vinegar, divided
floor soap
bucket of water

1. Add 1 cup vinegar to bucket of soapy water.

2. Wash floor; empty bucket and fill with water and 1 cup vinegar.

3. Rinse floors with vinegar water.

Floor Cleaner
(White Vinegar)

1/2 cup vinegar
1/4 cup liquid soap
1/4 cup lemon juice
2 gallons water

1. Combine all ingredients in a clean bucket.

2. Use on floors that need cleaned and brightened.

Carpet Stains
(White Vinegar)

1/2 cup vinegar
2 tablespoons salt

1. Combine ingredients until a soft paste forms.

2. Rub paste into carpet stain and dry completely (it is very important to allow paste to fully dry).

3. Vacuum up stain and chalky residue.

Carpet Stains, Heavy
(White Vinegar)

1/2 cup vinegar
2 tablespoons salt
2 tablespoons borax

1. Dissolve salt and borax in vinegar.

2. Rub solution into heavily soiled carpet stain and allow to dry completely (it is very important to allow this paste to fully dry).

3. Vacuum up stain and chalky residue.

Carpet Cleaning
(White Vinegar)

As with any new cleaning endeavor, be sure to test a small area of the carpet for colorfastness prior to cleaning larger areas.

1 cup vinegar
1 gallon water

1. Combine vinegar and water and pour into a spray bottle.

2. Spray carpet in areas that need cleaned and allow to soak in for several minutes.

3. Wipe clean with an absorbent cloth or towel.

4. If necessary repeat a second time, doing so before carpet has had an opportunity to dry.

Carpet Water Stains
(White Vinegar)

This is an excellent formula to remove stained carpet that has gotten wet, and left a stain from its own backing.

1/4 cup vinegar
1 cup water

1. Combine vinegar and water together.

2. Wet the stain with vinegar and water combination.

3. Blot dry with a paper towel or clean rag.

4. Repeat, if necessary.

Furniture: Polish
(White Vinegar)

1/8 cup vinegar
1/4 cup linseed oil
1/8 cup whiskey

1. Combine ingredients together in a small bowl.

2. Use to wipe and polish furniture with a soft cloth.

3. Allow alcohol to evaporate as solution air dries.

Furniture: Polish
(White Vinegar)

3/4 cup vinegar
1/4 cup lemon oil

1. Combine ingredients and store in a jar with a tight-fitting lid.

2. Use to polish furniture by wiping to a shine with a clean, soft cloth.

Furniture: Cleaner and Polish
(White Vinegar)

1/2 cup vinegar
1/2 cup olive oil

1. Combine both ingredients and pour into a jar with a fitted lid.

2. Use clean cloth to wipe solution onto wood furniture and buff dry.

Furniture: Wood Scratches
(White Vinegar)

2 tablespoons vinegar
2 tablespoons iodine
small artist brush

1. Combine ingredients together in a small dish.

2. Using brush, paint mixture deep into scratches, and allow to air dry.

3. For light colored scratches, add more vinegar; for dark colored scratches, add more iodine.

Furniture: Cleaning Wood Surfaces
(White Vinegar)

1 teaspoon vinegar
1 cup warm water

1. Combine vinegar and water in a small bowl.

2. Carefully wash down wood surfaces to prevent haze build up from commercial cleaners.

3. Buffing in a circular motion as you dry.

Furniture: Wood Paneling
(White Vinegar)

1 tablespoon vinegar
1 tablespoon olive oil
1 cup warm water

1. Mix all ingredients well in a small bowl.

2. Using a clean cloth, wipe down wood paneling to perk up appearance and restore shine.

Waxed Surfaces
(White Vinegar)

They key to washing waxed surfaces is to use cool water, instead of warm. Warm water softens the wax coating making it easier for tiny particles of dirt and dust to become embedded, dulling its shine.

1/2 cup vinegar
small bucket of cool water

1. Add vinegar to small bucket of cool water.

2. Wash down waxed surfaces with a clean rag soaked in vinegar solution.

3. Dry with a clean cloth.

Bathroom: Shower Head
(White Vinegar)

vinegar, undiluted
paper towels
plastic bag
rubber band
scrub brush

1. Soak paper towels in vinegar until saturated.

2. Wrap saturated paper towels tightly against shower head; do not wring out towels.

3. Place plastic bag around coated shower head and secure with a rubber band; set overnight.

4. In the morning, remove bag and paper towels and discard.

5. Wet scrub brush with additional vinegar and brush away any remaining mineral scales.

Bathroom: Shower Head
(White Vinegar)

1/2 cup vinegar
2/3 cup water

1. Combine vinegar and water.

2. Use soft cleaning brush to scrub clean mineral buildup on bathroom shower heads.

Bathroom: Shower Head
(White Vinegar)

vinegar, undiluted
hot rinse water
cleaning brush
toothpick or nail
toothbrush

1. Unscrew shower head and place in sink with enough undiluted vinegar to cover shower head.

2. Allow to soak for at least 30 minutes, more if necessary.

3. Remove shower head and gently brush with a cleaning brush.

4. Use toothpick or nail to clean out small openings, if blocked.

5. Scrub around openings with an old toothbrush.

6. Rinse in hot water.

7. Dry to a shine with a buffing towel.

Bathroom: Shower Curtains
(White Vinegar)

2 cups vinegar
warm water to cover curtain
2 tablespoons liquid detergent

1. Remove shower curtain from hooks and place in bathtub or wash tub.

2. Fill tub with just enough water to completely cover shower curtain.

3. Pour in 2 cups of vinegar.

4. Allow shower curtain to soak in vinegar water at least 4 hours, or overnight.

5. In the morning, add liquid detergent to vinegar water and wash curtain.

6. Hang outside in the afternoon sun to dry.

Bathroom: Chrome and Brass
(White Vinegar)

1/2 cup vinegar
2 cups warm water
wax

1. In sink or small bucket, combine vinegar and water.

2. Using a soft cloth, clean chrome and brass.

3. Dry completely.

4. Apply two coats of a light wax to coat and shine.

5. Coating will make future clean up easier and prevent buildup of hard water deposits.

Bathroom: Toilet Stains
(White Vinegar)

1 cup vinegar
1 cup borax

1. Pour vinegar over stained porcelain toilet.

2. Sprinkle borax over wet vinegar stain.

3. Let soak for 2 hours.

4. Brush with a toilet brush and flush away.

Bathroom: Glass Shower Doors
(White Vinegar)

1/4 cup vinegar
1 teaspoon alum

1. Mix two ingredients together.

2. Wipe mixture on glass shower door and scrub with a soft cleaning brush.

3. Rinse with hot water.

4. Buff with a soft cloth until completely dry.

Bathroom: Exhaust Fans
(White Vinegar)

vinegar, undiluted

1. Wipe and clean exhaust fan grill cover, removing dust and debris.

2. Using a clean cloth wet with vinegar, wipe down grill cover coating it with vinegar to keep dust from accumulating on fan grill.

Bathroom: Shower Door Mildew
(White Vinegar)

vinegar, undiluted
water
old toothbrush
cleaning cloth
spray bottle

1. Dip old toothbrush into undiluted vinegar; use to scrub out corners and crevices of shower door.

2. Use spray bottle filled with vinegar to wet shower door.

3. Wipe clean with a cloth saturated in water.

Bathroom: Soap Film Removal
(White Vinegar)

1/2 cup vinegar, plus 1/4 cup vinegar
1 cup baking soda
water

1. In a bowl, combine vinegar and baking soda into a creamy paste (add additional vinegar, if needed).

2. Spread creamy paste over soap film in shower and allow to set for 5 minutes.

3. Use a soft brush to clean film.

4. Rinse with warm bucket of water to which 1/4 cup vinegar has been added.

5. Use soft cloth to buff dry.

Bathroom: Soap Scum Removal
(White Vinegar)

1/2 cup vinegar, divided
1/4 cup ammonia
3 tablespoons baking soda

1. Combine 1/2 cup vinegar, ammonia and baking soda, and stir into a thick paste.

2. Spread mixture over soap scum.

3. Allow to set for at least 10 minutes.

4. Gently scrub with a cleaning brush.

5. Rinse with a bucket of cool water to which 1/4 cup additional vinegar has been added.

6. After removing soap scum from showers and doors, use Soap Film Preventative below to keep from returning.

Bathroom: Soap Film Preventative
(White Vinegar)

1 cup vinegar
1 quart water
spray bottle

1. Fill spray bottle with vinegar and water.

2. Once a week, spray down shower and tub area to prevent soap film from building up.

Bathroom: Odors
(White Vinegar)

1 tablespoon vinegar
1/2 cup water
small spray bottle

1. Fill spray bottle with vinegar and water.

2. Use a few sprays of this natural deodorizer in the place of aerosol air fresheners.

Bathroom: Ceramic Tile
(White Vinegar)

1/4 cup vinegar
1 cup water

1. Combine vinegar and water.

2. Use cloth or sponge to wipe down ceramic tile in the bathroom to keep soap scum and hard water salts from building up.

3. Dry thoroughly with a clean towel.

Mirrors
(White Vinegar)

vinegar, undiluted
soft, clean cloth

1. Spray vinegar directly onto clean cloth.

2. Use cloth to wipe mirror into a streak-free shine.

3. Do no spray vinegar, or any other solution, directly onto mirror. Moisture can make its way into silver backing and destroy mirror.

Streak-Free Window Cleaner
(White Vinegar)

1/4 cup vinegar
1 quart water
spray bottle

1. Combine all ingredients in a plastic spray bottle.

2. Spray onto windows and mirrors.

3. Wipe immediately with a soft cloth or paper towel.

All-Purpose Cleaner
(White Vinegar)

1/4 cup vinegar
2 cups water
3 tablespoons liquid detergent
plastic spray bottle

1. Fill spray bottle with all ingredients.

2. Great all-purpose cleaner for high dust areas, like banisters and window baseboards, etc.

Deep Window Cleaner
(White Vinegar)

1/4 cup vinegar
1/4 cup cornstarch

1. Combine ingredients together and dab thick solution onto dirty windows.

2. Allow to dry to a chalky film.

3. Rub off with a soft cloth in circular motion.

Household Window Cleaning Cloth
(White Vinegar)

1/4 cup vinegar
1/2 teaspoon liquid soap
2 cups water

1. Combine all ingredients together in a bowl.

2. Using a cloth, dip into mixture and wring out.

3. Store damp coated cloth in a glass jar with tight fitting lid.

4. Wipe spots from windows and mirrors as needed.

Windows: Drapery
(Apple Cider Vinegar)

This is a wonderful formula to freshen up drapery from existing odors and add a new freshness to the room. Be sure your drapes are free of heavy dust before wetting (dust can be easily eliminated with tools from your vacuum cleaner)

1 tablespoon vinegar
2 cups warm water
spray bottle

1. In a plastic bottle, combine warm water and vinegar; shake gently to combine.

2. Spritz each drapery panel and moisten drapes, paying particular attention to add a little extra solution to any wrinkles.

3. Allow to air dry, still hanging on the windows.

4. Drapes will smell fresher, and most of the wrinkles will disappear.

Windows: Fiberglass Drapes
(White Vinegar)

Fiberglass drapes demand special attention when getting cleaned. Try this formula to clean fiberglass drapes, while still keeping their delicate integrity.

1 tablespoon vinegar
2 cups water
plastic spray bottle
garden hose
outdoor clothesline

1. Hang drapes firmly on a clothesline and spray gently with a hose, fully wetting drapes.

2. Fill plastic spray bottle with water and vinegar.

3. Spray drapes with vinegar solution and allow to dry on clothesline for ultimate freshness.

Windows: Shutters and Louvered Doors
(White Vinegar)

Vinegar, undiluted
spray bottle
Paint stirring stick or ruler
soft clean cloth

1. Fill a spray bottle with undiluted vinegar.

2. Wrap a soft clean cloth around a paint stirring stick or ruler.

3. Spray cloth with vinegar and run it over and beneath each louver to get rid of dust.

Wallpaper Stripping
(White Vinegar)

1 cup vinegar
1 tablespoon liquid detergent
spray bottle

1. Combine vinegar and detergent in a spray bottle.

2. Wet wallpaper surface with vinegar solution and allow to set for 5 minutes.

3. Gently remove wallpaper with scraper, adding more solution as you go.

4. For difficult jobs, try "etching" wallpaper first, with a scoring tool; then wet wallpaper with solution and allow to set for another 5 minutes.

5. Wallpaper should now peel or scrape free.

Walls
(White Vinegar)

2 cups vinegar, divided
bucket warm water
few drops dish detergent

1. Combine all ingredients in a bucket.

2. Using a clean rag, wipe walls and allow to air dry.

3. For markings on wall that do not seem to wipe away, try a quick rub with undiluted vinegar.

4. Fill bucket with warm rinse water.

5. Add another cup of vinegar.

6. Use this solution with a clean cloth to rinse walls.

Ceilings
(White Vinegar)

1/2 cup vinegar
1 tablespoon dish detergent
half bucket of warm water

1. Combine all ingredients in a bucket.

2. In sections, use sponge or cloth to wash; drying each section before you begin a new.

3. A new paint roller brush on an extended broom handle works well for this, too.

Office: Bookshelves
(White Vinegar)

2 cups vinegar
bucket warm water
few drops liquid detergent

1. Add vinegar, water and a few drops of liquid detergent to bucket.

2. Using a rag or sponge, wipe down bookshelves, being certain to get into corners and crevices.

Office: Books
(White Vinegar)

1 tablespoon vinegar
2 cups water
fine mist spray bottle

1. Using a fine mist spray bottle, spray a soft cloth with this weak vinegar solution.

2. Use cloth to wipe books and dry immediately.

Office: Correction Fluid
(White Vinegar)

vinegar, undiluted

1. Dab area of furniture or cushion that has unwanted correction fluid.

2. Gently wipe with a paper towel to clean.

3. If spot is persistent, slightly saturate stain and blot away.

Office: Super Glue on Fingers
(White Vinegar)

vinegar, undiluted
small bowl

1. Fill a small bowl with undiluted vinegar.

2. Soak affected fingers for several minutes.

3. Peel away stuck on glue.

Office: Construction Paper Stains
(White Vinegar)

Colored construction paper, when it becomes wet, can leave colored stains on desks and other furniture. Try this formula for simple and thorough removal.

1/4 cup vinegar
1/4 cup water

1. Combine both vinegar and water together.

2. Use paper towel to blot up wet construction paper stains.

Nursery: High Chair Cleaning
(White Vinegar)

vinegar, undiluted
spray bottle
cleaning cloth

1. Set high chair in the shower and spray with full strength vinegar.

2. Allow to set for 5 minutes.

3. Turn shower on with warm water and spray high chair for 3 minutes.

4. Wipe food and grime off chair.

5. Give a final rinse and wipe dry.

Nursery: Odors
(White Vinegar)

This is a great, noninvasive method for eliminating odor from baby's nursery.

vinegar, undiluted
spray bottle
damp towel taken from washing machine

1. Take a clean towel that has just been washed, but still damp, from the washing machine.

2. Spray damp towel with vinegar and hang over door in baby's room.

3. As towel dries it will work to control odors and add clean moisture to the room.

Nursery: Baby Bottle Nipples
(White Vinegar)

1 teaspoon vinegar
2 cups water

1. In a clean pan, add vinegar and water together, and drop in baby bottle nipples.

2. Bring to a boil and continue boiling for several minutes.

3. This will not only clean and sterilize nipples, but also keep them from developing a sour taste.

Nursery: Toys
(White Vinegar)

1/4 cup vinegar
1 cup water

1. In a small bowl, combine vinegar and water.

2. Use this solution to wipe down baby toys, plastic dolls, blocks and blocks.

Children and Babies: Toys
(White Vinegar)

1/4 cup vinegar
1 quart hot water
few drops of soap

1. Combine all ingredients in a bowl or small tub.

2. Use to wash down baby's toys.

3. Rinse well and dry.

Play Clay for Children
(White Vinegar)

Here is a great, non-toxic recipe for play clay that is completely natural and safe for children to use.

1 teaspoon vinegar
1 cup flour
1/2 cup salt
1 cup water
1 teaspoon vinegar
1 tablespoon oil
food coloring, if desired

1. Combine all ingredients in a saucepan over medium heat.

2. Stir continually until it forms into a ball.

3. Remove from heat and allow to cool.

4. Knead clay ball until smooth.

5. Add a few drops of food coloring, if desired.

6. Store in a tightly sealed container or wrapped in plastic wrap in the refrigerator.

Air Freshener
(White Vinegar)

1 tablespoon vinegar
1 teaspoon baking soda
2 cups water
spray bottle

1. Combine ingredients in a plastic spray bottle.

2. Spray into the air in rooms needing a freshening up.

Odors: Room Deodorizer
(Apple Cider Vinegar)

1 cup vinegar
1/4 cup water
1 tablespoon cinnamon

1. Heat vinegar and water on stove top until hot.

2. Remove from heat and pour into a bowl.

3. Sprinkle cinnamon on top of vinegar solution

4. Place bowl on a low table in room to be freshened.

Painting: Odor-Free Painting
(Either Type)

3 cups vinegar, divided

1. Fill three small bowls with 1 cup vinegar in each bowl.

2. Place around room being painted to help absorb fresh paint odors while painting.

Painting: Concrete Walls and Floors
(White Vinegar)

This formula will help prep concrete walls and floors for painting, cutting down on peeling.

vinegar, undiluted
brush or roller

1. Brush or paint on undiluted vinegar as a preparation for walls about to be pained.

2. Allow to air dry before beginning to paint.

Painting: Remove Old Paint from Wood Windows
(White Vinegar)

1/2 cup vinegar
1/2 cup liquid detergent
paintbrush
razor blade or scraper

1. Combine vinegar and liquid detergent and mix.

2. Use a paintbrush to brush vinegar mixture onto wood that needs paint removed.

3. Soak for 5 minutes, then begin to carefully scrape away old paint with a razor or scraper.

Painted Surfaces: Wash
(White Vinegar)

1/4 cup vinegar
1 tablespoon cornstarch
2 cups hot water

1. Combine ingredients in a bowl or storage cup.

2. Wipe (or spray) solution on painted surface.

3. Immediately dry with a clean cloth (do not allow solution to soak into paint).

Misc: Ashtrays
(White Vinegar)

1/8 cup vinegar
1/8 cup hot water

1. Combine vinegar and hot water.

2. Fill ashtray and allow to sit overnight to get rid of lingering smoke odors.

Misc: Hairbrushes
(White Vinegar)

1/2 cup vinegar
2 cups hot water
2-3 drops liquid soap

1. Mix vinegar, water and a few drops of liquid soap.

2. Immerse hairbrushes in vinegar solution.

3. Let stand for 30 minutes.

4. Rinse hairbrushes clean and allow to air dry.

Misc: Hairbrushes, Combs and Rollers
(White Vinegar)

1 cup vinegar, plus 1/4 cup vinegar
1 quart warm water, plus extra water
few drops liquid detergent
old toothbrush

1. Combine 1 cup vinegar and warm water in a large bowl or sink basin.

2. Place brushes, combs and rollers in vinegar water and allow to soak for one hour.

3. Remove items and brush away any lingering build up with old toothbrush to which a few drops of liquid detergent has been added.

4. Rinse with clear water.

5. Refill sink basin with clean warm water and add 1/4 cup more vinegar.

6. Use this vinegar water to rinse brushes and combs clean one last time.

Misc: Eyeglasses
(White Vinegar)

1 tablespoon vinegar
cotton ball or soft cloth

1. Drench cotton ball or soft cloth with vinegar.

2. Wipe eyeglasses and allow to air dry, streak-free.

Misc: Moth Repellent
(White Vinegar)

1/2 cup vinegar
1/4 cup lavender
small cloth or sachet

1. Combine vinegar and lavender in a small jar.

2. Leave jar open in moth-ridden areas; also saturate small clothes or sachets with this solution, and place in areas you wish to rid of moths.

Misc: Moth Repellent
(White Vinegar)

2 cups vinegar
1/2 cup lavender leaves

1. Heat vinegar over stove top and add torn lavender leaves.

2. Simmer 10 minutes, and remove from heat.

3. Allow to cool.

4. Pour into jar with a tight fitting lid.

5. Allow to steep for 10 days.

6. Use to wipe down walls and plastic storage bins in clothes closet to drive away moths.

Misc: Silk House Plants
(White Vinegar)

1/4 cup vinegar
1 quart water

1. Combine both ingredients in a small bowl.

2. Use paper towel or cleaning rag to dab in solution and wipe dust and dirt from silk and plastic house plants.

3. Allow to air dry.

4. You can also pour this solution into a plastic spray bottle and use to spray silk plants to keep dust from forming.

Misc: Ballpoint Pen Stains
(White Vinegar)

vinegar, undiluted
clean cloth

1. Wet area stained with ballpoint pen with vinegar. You can do this by drizzling vinegar over the area and allow to penetrate if stained area is cloth; for areas that are vertical, soak a clean cloth in vinegar and drape cloth over stain.

2. Allow to soak in for 10 to 15 minutes.

3. Blot up with clean cloth.

4. Repeat, if necessary.

5. Thoroughly dry when finished.

Misc: Lamp Shades
(White Vinegar)

2 cups vinegar, divided
3 tablespoons liquid detergent
bucket or small tub of hot water

1. Combine vinegar and liquid detergent in bucket of hot water.

2. Take old lamp shade and immerse one corner of shade in tub of water, and move it around vigorously to clean.

3. Take shade out, turn it to a different corner and repeat until entire shade has been cleaned.

4. Remove shade from water and empty tub.

5. Refill tub with clean water and add another cup of vinegar.

6. Repeat same clean and shake motion to now rinse lampshade.

7. Allow to air dry.

Misc: Chewing Gum
(White Vinegar)

vinegar; undiluted, enough to cover gum

1. Soak chewing gum in undiluted vinegar.

2. Soak until chewing gum begins to dissolve.

3. If chewing gum will not dissolve, repeat above steps with heated vinegar.

Misc: Sticker or Decal Remover
(White Vinegar)

vinegar; undiluted
cotton ball or paper towel

1. Wet a cotton ball or paper towel with vinegar; sticker or decal should be saturated.

2. Soak until sticker or decal can be removed.

3. Repeat if necessary until sticker and glue residue comes free.

4. For stickers or decals that will not come free, gently scratch the top layer off, or scratch grooves into the paper.

5. Then, repeat steps above, allowing to soak until sticker or decal will break free.

Misc: Glass or Plastic Bead Jewelry
(White Vinegar)

1 tablespoon vinegar
2 quarts warm water, divided
1 teaspoon liquid detergent

1. Combine 1 quart of water and liquid detergent.

2. Dip strand of glass or plastic beads into water.

3. Remove from water and immediately dip into second bowl in which 1 quart of water and vinegar has been added to rinse clean.

4. Blot dry with a paper towel and complete drying with hair dryer on lowest setting.

Misc: Urine Stained Mattress
(White Vinegar)

This formula will not only remove unsightly urine stains from mattresses, but also the unpleasant odor that accompanies it.

vinegar, undiluted
spray bottle
soft cloths or paper towels

1. Spray urine stained area of mattress with undiluted vinegar.

2. Allow to set for 2 – 3 minutes.

3. Use a cloth or paper towel to blot dry.

4. May need to repeat process until entire stain comes clean.

Misc: Wet Dry Vac
(White Vinegar)

Wet Dry Vacs tend to smell musty after time. Try using this formula periodically to freshen vac and extend the life of this appliance.

1 cup vinegar
2 quarts warm water

1. Combine vinegar and warm water together.

2. Suck up solution in vac and set for 5 minutes.

3. Empty machine and wipe out inside of the vac.

4. Allow wet vac to air dry completely before putting it back together for storage.

Misc: Denture Cleaner
(Either Type)

You can also add a tablespoon of fresh mint leaves, torn into pieces, to this formula for a fresh twist.

1 teaspoon vinegar
1 cup water

1.   Add vinegar to cup of water.

2.   Place dentures in vinegar water and allow to soak overnight.

Fireplace Ashes
(White Vinegar)

Vinegar water solution keeps ashes from flying around the room and help neutralize alkali in the ash.

2 tablespoons vinegar
2 cups water
spray bottle

1.   Fill spray bottle with water and vinegar.

2.   Before scooping out ashes, spray them down with a coating of vinegar and water solution.

3.   Now scoop out wet ashes (this will help keep them from flying all over the room).

4.   Continue to spray as you clean to keep dust and ash particles to a minimum.

5.   When finished scooping out ashes, use remaining vinegar solution to thoroughly clean fireplace if finished using for the season.

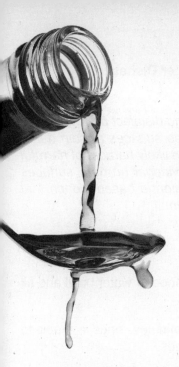

Chapter Seven

Pets and the Great Outdoors

Let's not confine vinegar's usefulness to just inside our home. Vinegar's amazing power extends well beyond the borders of your house and makes an ideal choice for outdoor projects as well. Make vinegar your choice as a natural degreaser, insect repelling agent, and antibacterial cleaner and disinfectant. Vinegar is completely natural and safe enough to eat, and is ideal to use in vegetable gardens and on fruit bushes and trees. It is useful in the garden, as it helps deter insects and promote better soil pH levels for growing vegetables and other plants.

And why stop with just our yards and gardens? Vinegar is the perfect option for pet care, as it is a gentle, yet powerful anti-odor, anti-bacterial solution.

With vinegar being an environmentally safe substance, completely biodegradable and non-damaging to riverbeds and streams, one would be hard pressed to find a more ideal product for outdoor applications.

So grab a bottle or two of vinegar, and let's head out into the great outdoors!

Pets: Clean Food and Water Dishes
(White Vinegar)

Try this formula to clean and disinfect pets' food and water bowls. Because these surfaces remain damp throughout the day, they are likely harbors of harmful bacteria and mold. Using vinegar on pets' surfaces avoids the need to use chlorine based bleach that might be harmful to the animal.

1/4 cup vinegar
water

1. Pour vinegar into pet's food or water bowl and fill with water.

2. Allow to soak for 20 minutes, once a week to clean and disinfect dishes.

Pets: Ticks
(Apple Cider Vinegar)

Try this formula on your hunting dog prior to heading outdoors.

vinegar, undiluted
1/2 cup chamomile flowers

1. Combine vinegar and chamomile flowers in a small bowl.

2. Set for 15 minutes to allow flower to thoroughly mix into vinegar.

3. Wipe this mixture into dog's coat, or onto cat's fur to discourage ticks.

Pets: Flea Elimination in Home
(White Vinegar)

1/2 cup vinegar
1/4 cup water
1 tablespoon fennel

1. Combine all ingredients and pour into a spray bottle.

2. Thoroughly saturate areas where pets sleep or play with vinegar solution.

3. Allow to air dry.

Pets: Fleas on Pets
(White Vinegar)

1 cup vinegar
1 tablespoon rue, chopped

1. Combine vinegar and rue in a small bowl.

2. Rub this combination into dog's hair to discourage or get rid of nasty fleas.

Pets: Long Haired Cats
(White Vinegar)

3 tablespoons vinegar
1 quart water

1. Combine together vinegar and warm water.

2. After bathing cat, rinse long fur in this vinegar solution.

3. Fur will shine and mats will brush out easier.

Pet Hair
(White Vinegar)

Remove pet hair on furniture, carpet or clothing.

vinegar, undiluted
spray bottle
discarded sock

1. Turn an old tube sock inside out and slip it over your hand.

2. Spray it lightly with vinegar.

3. Use dampened sock to wipe down furniture, carpet or clothing to remove pet hair.

4. Dampened sock can also be used to wipe down pet directly, removing fallen hair.

Pets: Urine Stains
(White Vinegar)

vinegar, undiluted
1 tablespoon baking soda
Spray bottle
Scrub brush

1. If urine stains are still damp, blot with towel.

2. Using vinegar in a spray bottle, completely dampen area of urine stain.

3. Sprinkle baking soda over dampened stain.

4. Using a scrub brush, brush stained area in a circular motion.

5. Allow to dry completely.

6. When dry, vacuum up stain and residue.

Pets: Urine
(White Vinegar)

vinegar, undiluted
Spray bottle
Paper towels

1. Blot up excess urine with paper towels.

2. Spray white vinegar over entire area that has been affected.

3. Blot up vinegar liquid.

4. Repeat again, as necessary.

Pets: Behavior Issues
(Either Type)

This is a great, easy solution to solving unwanted pet problems.

1 teaspoon vinegar
few tablespoons water
squirt gun

1. Fill squirt gun with water, leaving a small amount of room.

2. Add vinegar.

3. When pet approaches a forbidden area, or begins to engage in unwanted behavior such as scratching or chewing, tell them a stern "No" and reinforce it with a quick liquid reminder. Soon, simply picking up the squirt gun will ensure good behavior.

Pets: Dog Itching
(Apple Cider Vinegar)

1/3 cup vinegar
2 quarts warm water

1. Shampoo and rinse dog as usual.

2. Combine ingredients and pour over dog; do not rinse.

3. Dry dog as usual and coat will be shiny and soft, cutting down on itching and scratching.

Pets: Dog Odor
(White Vinegar)

Make a bottle full of this mixture to keep on hand for daily odor control of all furry pets.

2 tablespoons vinegar
2 cups water
spray bottle

1. Pour vinegar and water in a large spray bottle.

2. Spray coat daily to help eliminate odor.

Pets: Jellyfish Stings
(Either Type)

Keep this formula in mind when taking your dog on vacation.

vinegar, undiluted

1. At first notice of jellyfish sting, pour undiluted vinegar over sting area to help dilute the poison.

Pets: Shiny Horse's Coat
(Apple Cider Vinegar)

1/8 cup vinegar, undiluted

1. Pour vinegar into horse's water trough daily to keep his coat shiny and healthy.

Aquariums
(White Vinegar)

Spray vinegar onto cloth, not directly on aquarium glass. Tiny droplets may get into aquarium and upset delicate pH balance, possibly harming fish.

1 teaspoon vinegar
1 cup water
spray bottle
clean cloth

1. Mix vinegar and water in a plastic spray bottle.

2. Spray soft cloth with vinegar solution and wipe clean aquarium exterior; buff dry.

3. If aquarium exterior is extremely dirty, use undiluted vinegar and wipe clean.

Birdbaths
(White Vinegar)

Use this formula to control growth of fungus and bacteria in outdoor bird baths.

2 tablespoons vinegar

1. Add vinegar to outdoor birdbath water every time you fill up the bird bath.

Insects: Mosquitoes
(White Vinegar)

2 cups vinegar
1/2 cup lavender flowers

1. Warm vinegar on stove and add lavender flowers.

2. Simmer for 10 minutes.

3. Cool, and pour into a bowl or jar.

4. Sprinkle around yard to keep mosquitoes at bay.

Insects: Fleas
(White Vinegar)

2 cups vinegar
1/2 cup basil, torn

1. Combine vinegar and torn basil leaves together and warm on the stove top.

2. Simmer for 20 minutes.

3. Cool completely.

4. Pour in a thick line along home's doorways to prevent fleas from entering the house.

Insects: Fire Ant Hills
(White Vinegar)

vinegar, undiluted

1. Saturate ant hills with undiluted vinegar to get rid of fire ants.

2. May need to repeat, making sure vinegar is working its way down into the ant hill.

Insects: Ants
(White Vinegar)

vinegar, undiluted
spray bottle

1. Fill a spray bottle with undiluted vinegar.

2. Use to spray cupboards and countertops to rid home of ants.

Garden Insects: Aphids
(White Vinegar)

2 cups vinegar
1 cup mint leaves, shredded

1. Combine vinegar and shredded mint leaves, an allow to set for 10 minutes.

2. Wet a circle of ground around cabbage, Brussels sprouts and cauliflower plants with this mint vinegar mixture to keep aphids from dining on plants.

Garden Insects: Flying Insects
(White Vinegar)

1/4 cup vinegar
2 bay leaves, crushed
spray bottle

1. Pour vinegar into plastic spray bottle.

2. Crush bay leaves and add to vinegar.

3. Spray down picnic table and outlying area to keep flies and other insects at bay.

Garden Insects: Cucumber and Melon Plants
(White Vinegar)

2 cups vinegar
1/4 cup oregano leaves

1. Combine vinegar and oregano together, and allow to set for at least 15 minutes.

2. Wet ground area around cucumber or melon plants every week to keep bugs from eating plants.

Garden Insects: Vegetables
(White Vinegar)

2 cups vinegar
1/4 cup sage, chopped

1. Combine vinegar and sage together, and store in a plastic bottle.

2. Sprinkle sage vinegar around vegetable vines to keep plant-eating insects away.

Garden Insects: Tomatoes
(White Vinegar)

1 cup vinegar
1/4 cup basil leaves, chopped

1. Combine vinegar and chopped basil leaves, and allow to set for at least 15 minutes.

2. Soak ground beneath tomato plants to keep insects away.

Garden: Balance pH Soil Level
(White Vinegar)

1 cup vinegar
bucket of water

1. Pour vinegar into bucket of clean water.

2. Pour in a circle around acid loving plants, such as azaleas, blueberries, marigolds and radishes.

Garden: Paths and Stones
(Apple Cider Vinegar)

1/2 cup vinegar
1 tablespoon fresh thyme

1. Combine ingredients together.

2. Sprinkle or spray onto garden paths and stepping stones as a wonderful pest repellent.

3. This concoction will also help keep mold and mildew from forming on stones.

Garden: Clay Flowerpots
(White Vinegar)

Mineral deposits not only make the pots appear unsightly, but can also interfere with the way clay pots breathe and absorb water.

vinegar, undiluted
scrub brush
clean water

1. Dip scrub brush in vinegar and scrub outside of pots; if pot is empty, also clean the inside.

2. Use fresh water to rinse the pot clean.

Garage: Cement Floor
(White Vinegar)

Use this simple formula to clean a dirty garage floor.

1 cup vinegar
1 gallon water
shredded newspaper

1. In a bucket, add vinegar to a gallon of water.

2. Take a pile of shredded newspaper, and pour vinegar water over.

3. Toss wet shredded newspaper over garage floor, and sweep with a push broom.

4. Dust will cling to the newspaper and the vinegar is used to help neutralize odors.

Garage: Cement Floor
(Apple Cider Vinegar)

This will give you a second use for grass clippings, as you clean dust and debris from garage floor.

1 cup vinegar
grass clippings

1. Use grass clippings to spread around garage floor.

2. Sprinkle vinegar over clippings and allow to set for 5 – 10 minutes.

3. Using a push broom, sweep flooring clean.

4. Garage will not only look clean, but also smell fresh.

Garage: Cement Floor Oil Stains
(White Vinegar)

This formula is excellent to remove oil stains from a leaky car engine.

1 cup vinegar
1/2 gallon water
1 -2 cups dry laundry detergent

1. Soak up as much standing oil as possible with paper towels.

2. Sprinkle a heavy coat of dry laundry detergent over oil stain and allow to absorb.

3. Using a push broom, brush away oil that has now collected on detergent.

4. Repeat, if necessary.

5. Add vinegar to water in a bucket.

6. Pour over old stained area and spray out with a garden hose.

Garage: Clean Tools
(White Vinegar)

1/4 cup vinegar
1 quart water

1. Combine both ingredients in a small bowl.

2. Use mixture to clean away mineral buildup on metal tools.

Garage: Clean Paintbrushes
(White Vinegar)

1 quart vinegar

1. Pour vinegar into pot along with dirty paintbrushes. Bring to a boil.

2. Cover pot and remove from stove; let set for one hour.

3. Place vinegar pot with brushes back on stove top and bring to a gentle boil again.

4. Simmer for 20 minutes.

5. Rinse brushes well, working the softened paint out of the bristles with your fingers.

6. For extremely have paint encrustations, repeat the process a second time.

Window Screens
(White Vinegar)

1 cup vinegar
1/2 gallon water

1. Combine vinegar and water in a bucket.

2. Use sponge to clean dirty window screens.

3. For screens with heavy buildup, pretreat screens prior to cleaning by putting vinegar in a spray bottle and wetting screens first. Allow to sit with vinegar solution for ten minutes, then clean as usual.

Old Brooms, New Life
(Apple Cider Vinegar)

This is a great way to give a second life to an old, about-to-be-discarded broomstick.

1 cup vinegar
bucket of hot water
old, ragged broom
Knife or scissors

1. Using a knife or scissors, carefully cut about half the length of the broom's bristles off, but cutting it to a deep angle (leaving the short side about 1 inch in length, and the longer side about 6 inches in length).

2. Add vinegar to bucket of hot water and soak newly cut broom for about 15 minutes.

3. Remove broom and shake, getting rid of most of the excess liquid.

4. Set broom in sun to air dry.

5. When completely dry, use this new angled broom to reach hard to clean floor corners.

Air Conditioner Grills
(White Vinegar)

vinegar, undiluted
clean cloth

1. Wipe away dirt and debris from air conditioner grills as usual.

2. Using a clean cloth or rag, wipe grill with undiluted vinegar to inhibit future dust buildup.

Barbecue Grills
(White Vinegar)

2 cups vinegar
2 tablespoons dishwasher detergent
2 quarts hot water
plastic garbage bag
spray bottle
cleaning rag

1. Remove soiled barbecue rack from grill and place in plastic garbage bag.

2. Fill spray bottle with vinegar and use to wet down entire rack.

3. Tie garbage bag in a loose knot to seal in the moisture.

4. Place bag with rack in the warm sun and leave for 4 hours.

5. Untie bag (do not rip) and add dishwasher detergent and hot water.

6. Retie bag and leave rack to soak for an additional 2 hours.

7. Open bag and use cleaning rag to wipe rack.

Driveway: Grass in Cracks
(White Vinegar)

vinegar, undiluted

1. Pour vinegar over cracks in driveways or sidewalk where grass is growing in between blocks.

2. Repeat as necessary.

Car: Chrome
(White Vinegar)

vinegar, undiluted
Clean cloth

1. Wipe down car chrome with undiluted vinegar.

2. Buff dry to a high shine with soft cloth.

Car: Chrome Rust Spots
(White Vinegar)

vinegar, undiluted
aluminum foil
rinse water
wax

1. Tear off a small piece of foil and dip in vinegar.

2. Rub out small rust spots on chrome until they are completely gone.

3. Rinse away debris and dry completely with a clean towel.

4. Using a small amount of wax, add a thin wax coating to protect chrome and discourage new rust spots from forming.

Car: Window Interiors
(White Vinegar)

1/2 cup vinegar
1/4 cup water

1. Combine vinegar and water.

2. Use a paper towel or chamois to wipe finger-prints and smudges from windows.

Car: Ashtrays
(White Vinegar)

vinegar, undiluted
newspaper or paper towel

1. Wipe out dirty ashtray with wadded up newspaper or paper towel drenched in vinegar.

2. Allow to air dry; vinegar will neutralize the ashtray odor.

Car: Vinyl Interiors
(White Vinegar)

1/2 cup vinegar
1 teaspoons liquid soap
1/2 cup water

1. Combine all ingredients in a small bowl.

2. Wipe onto vinyl surfaces with a clean cloth.

3. Rinse with clear water and buff dry.

Car: Freshen Interior
(Apple Cider Vinegar)

Mix this solution in advance to keep on hand as an easy air freshener for cars. Trial-size spray bottles are perfect for this project.

1/4 cup vinegar
small, fine mist spray bottle

1. Fill fine mist spray bottle with undiluted vinegar.

2. Gently mist car interior for a fresh, clean smell.

Car: Windshield Washer Cleaner
(White Vinegar)

This windshield washer cleaner is excellent for a no-streak, no-freeze windshield cleaner.

1/2 cup vinegar
2 cups rubbing alcohol
1 tablespoon liquid detergent
6 cups water

1. In a small bucket, combine water and liquid detergent.

2. Add vinegar and alcohol and combine.

3. Pour into windshield washer reservoir.

Car: Bumper Sticker Removal
(White Vinegar)

vinegar, undiluted
cloth or small towel

1. Completely saturate cloth or small towel in vinegar; do not wring out.

2. Wrap soaked vinegar cloth around bumper where decal is attached.

3. All to set for 45 minutes.

4. Remove wet towel and pull of sticker.

5. Repeat, if necessary.

6. You may wish to use soaked towel to further wipe off any residual glue once sticker has been removed.

Boats: Stains and Discoloration
(White Vinegar)

Aluminum boats are extremely sensitive to alkaline in the water, which can etch aluminum and cause discoloration. Vinegar is an excellent source to neutralize alkaline, making it easier to scrub away discoloration.

vinegar, undiluted
clean water rinse

1. Using a towel saturated in vinegar, wipe clean any stains or discoloration appearing on boat.

2. Rinse clean with clear water.

3. Wipe dry.

Campers and RVs: Fiberglass
(White Vinegar)

vinegar, undiluted
spray bottle
rinse water
paper towel

1. Spray areas of fiberglass camper with undiluted vinegar where hard water has left stains.

2. Wipe down with cloth and dry completely.

3. For tough to clean stains, soak a paper towel in vinegar and "stick" on top of stain for 5 minutes.

4. Remove paper towel and wipe clean.

5. Rinse and dry completely.

Campers and RVs: Easy Laundry Cleaning
(White Vinegar)

No access to a laundry machine on the road? Try this novel, but functional, method for washing laundry while camping. Using this formula, a watertight container is used as a "washing machine" to launder clothing while you are driving (driving works to "agitate" laundry and clean clothing). You will arrive at your day's destination with clean clothes, ready to rinse and air dry.

1 cup vinegar
2-3 tablespoons laundry detergent
5 gallons water
watertight container

1. In watertight container, add vinegar, water and laundry detergent.

2. Place clothing in container and seal tightly.

3. Secure in camper and proceed on day's drive.

4. When you arrive at your destination, rinse with clean water and hang outside to dry.

Luggage: Odor
(White Vinegar)

1/4 cup vinegar
clean cloth

1. Wet cloth with vinegar and wring out excess.

2. Place damp cloth in luggage and close, but do not zipper shut.

3. Allow to set overnight.

Camping: Plastic Picnic Coolers
(White Vinegar)

2 cups vinegar, divided
1 teaspoon liquid detergent
1 gallon water, plus 1 cup water
extra water for rinsing

1. Empty plastic cooler and wipe out all food crumbs and debris.

2. Pour 1 cup vinegar, liquid detergent and 1 gallon of water.

3. Using a cleaning cloth, make sure solution soaks all areas of the cooler, including inside of the lid.

4. Put lid back onto cooler and allow to set while the outside of cooler is being cleaned.

5. To clean out side of cooler, combine second cup of vinegar and 1 cup water.

6. Use a cloth to wipe down cooler's exterior.

7. Open cooler and dump out contents.

8. Wipe down the inside and rinse thoroughly.

9. Dry entire cooler.

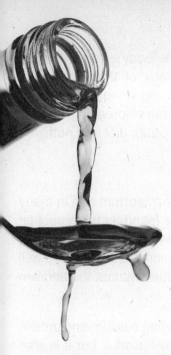

Chapter Eight

Cooking with Vinegar: Healthy from the Inside Out

Up to now, we have concentrated on using vinegar as either a home remedy ingredient, or as a potent cleaning agent. We have focused mainly on external uses, or on counteracting a problem once it has festered. Now it is time to focus on vinegar's hearty addition to a nutritious diet as a means of preventative medicine, or just to enjoy its robust taste!

What vinegar does for aches, pains and illness it can also do for better overall health. The same amazing vinegar that boasts so many vitamins and minerals as a natural healer, can work from the inside out to deliver better health and longevity by making this substance part of your healthy eating plan.

Packed with Nutrients for Healthy Living

As we discussed in chapter two, vinegar is naturally packed with nutrients essential for healthy living. Through time and neglect, the human body can become depleted of these important nutrients. So, as time goes on, this nutrient depletion can become more evident with the onset of noticeable health issues and obvious changes to skin and hair. By keeping the body's nutrient levels complete, some researchers believe many of these maladies can be avoided in the first place. While using vinegar as a home remedy can induce amazing results, the idea of foregoing many of those problems in the first place through better diet and nutrition, is even more amazing.

Easily and Tastily Added to the Menu

Did you know vinegar already plays an important role in many of the foods that we eat? Vinegar can be found as an ingredient in tomato catsup, salad dressings, pickles, sauces, mayonnaise, as well as a host of other foods and common entrees. It pairs well with vegetables and can add flavor to dishes without the addition of extra salt,

Vinegar is an excellent solution for adding calcium and protein to the diet. Not only is vinegar amazingly flavorful, but it is also widely used as a natural preservative, keeping foods fresher longer, and free from harmful bacteria.

Why Vinegar?

Even outside of its medicinal properties, scientific research shows vinegar is one of the best entities to include in a well-balanced diet. Still not convinced? Take a look at this list of vinegar's many culinary uses:

- Adds a host of body essentials to the diet, such as proteins, carbohydrates, vitamins and minerals.

- Vinegar's unique flavor, when combined with honey, can bring a sweet and sour touch to gourmet dishes.

- Vinegar's antibacterial properties help preserve food and lengthen shelf life.

- Vinegar come in not only apple or white vinegar, but also a host of flavored choices you can purchase or make yourself (see a few favorite recipes for flavored vinegar in this chapter).

- Vinegar can help keep homemade candy and frostings smooth and free from gritty sugar granules. Just add a few drops of white vinegar to the recipe.

- The acidic nature of vinegar, in combination with its robust flavor, makes it an obvious choice as a meat tenderizer, soften muscle fibers and bringing tenderness to even the toughest cuts of meat.

- Vinegar's acid also works to tenderize tough cellulose found in many vegetables such as beets, celery, spinach and cabbage, that make those foods tougher to digest.

- Placing a little white vinegar on white vegetables such as cauliflower gives them a beautiful bleaching effect. It also prevents enzymatic browning. Enzymatic browning is when foods tend to darken after exposure to air. This browning is often accompanied by an off-taste.

- When vinegar is added to fish dishes, I can help eliminate traditional fish odor. It also helps get rid of fish odor during clean up.

- Place a quick splash of white vinegar in the water as potatoes are boiling to help keep them snowy white.

- Using vinegar in soups or pastas, helps add robust flavor without the need for additional salt.

- As an added bonus, vinegar's sour and acidic taste stimulates saliva flow. This enhances the mouth's ability to taste and enjoy other food sensations.

Vinegar and Osteoporosis

Vinegar also has an amazing feature of being able to extract and convey nutrients from one food to another. For example, when chicken bones are cooked in vinegar, the calcium from the bones is extracted by the vinegar and released in the broth. Why is this important? Because osteoporosis is a major condition as we age. And calcium is a crucial factor in the prevention and fight of this bone crippling disease. So while vinegar is a healthy and delicious addition to the menu, it also goes a long way in the fight against osteoporosis.

With all these healthy reasons to enjoy vinegar, why not try adding a few of these delicious recipes to your home cookbook? Bon appétit and here's to healthy living!

Vinegar as a Preservative
(Apple Cider Vinegar)

vinegar, undiluted
spray bottle

1. Fill a plastic spray bottle with undiluted vinegar.

2. Spray down meat that will be stored for several days in the refrigerator to retard yeast, mold and bacteria growth and increasing its shelf life.

Calcium-Rich Salad
(Apple Cider Vinegar)

Any of your favorite greens work, such as baby spinach leaves, collard greens and kale.

2 tablespoons vinegar
2 cups favorite greens, torn
2 tablespoons honey
1 tablespoon water
1/4 cup feta cheese

1. Place torn greens in a serving bowl.

2. Combine vinegar, honey and water, and pour over greens.

3. Top with feta cheese and serve.

Vinegar Salad Dressing
(Apple Cider Vinegar)

1/4 cup vinegar
1/4 cup corn oil
1/8 cup honey

1. Combine all ingredients together.

2. Serve over fruits or vegetables to add vinegar to your diet.

Vinegar Salad Dressing
(Apple Cider Vinegar)

1/4 cup vinegar
1 teaspoon olive oil
1/8 cup honey

3. Combine all ingredients together.

4. Serve over a small bowl of greens.

Legumes and Vegetables
(Apple Cider Vinegar)

This formula will help make legumes more digestible, therefore having less painful gas.

1-2 tablespoons vinegar
favorite legumes or veggies

1. Add a splash of vinegar to legumes and vegetables as they begin to heat.

2. Cook as normal.

Chicken Soup
(Apple Cider Vinegar)

Enjoy this healthy low-calorie, calcium-rich soup. The vinegar works to pull extra calcium from the bones and into the soup!

1/2 cup vinegar
2-3 pounds chicken bones
3/4 cup pastina or other tiny pasta
2 bouillon cubes
2 slightly beaten egg whites
2 tablespoons chopped parsley
1 gallon water

1. Heat water and vinegar over medium heat until warm.

2. Simmer chicken bones for at least 2 hours, uncovered allowing steam to escape.

3. Strain the broth and skim off all fat.

4. Strip the meat from the bones, and add chicken, pasta and bouillon cubes to the stock.

5. Bring to a boil and cook for 10 minutes.

6. Remove from heat and add egg whites to soup, stirring constantly.

7. Mix in parsley and serve immediately.

Vegetable Beef Soup
(Apple Cider Vinegar)

Not fond of chicken soup, but still looking for a calcium-rich soup? Try this vegetable beef recipe!

1/2 cup vinegar
1 gallon water
2 pounds short ribs (prime rib roast works well)
medium onion, chopped
2 garlic cloves
1/4 cup fresh parsley
2-3 sprigs fresh rosemary
2 carrots, chopped
1 tomato, chopped (canned may also be used)
1/2 cup corn
1/2 cup green beans
1/2 cup garbanzo beans
1/2 cup barley
1/2 cup potatoes, cubed small
pinch of salt

1. In a large pot, place short ribs and cover with water and vinegar. Add chopped onion and garlic cloves.

2. Simmer gently on low heat for 3 hours.

3. Skim off the fat, and then strain the broth.

4. Add broth back to the pot along with two cups of small pieces of strained out beef chunks.

5. Add remaining ingredients and bring to a boil.

6. Continue boiling until potato cubes and carrots are tender.

7. Serve warm.

Garden Vegetable Wash
(White Vinegar)

1 cup vinegar
1 tablespoon salt
1 gallon water

1. Combine vinegar, salt and water in sink or large bowl.

2. Wash fresh garden vegetables in this solution to eliminate any garden pests or bugs prior to cooking.

Vinaigrette
(Apple Cider Vinegar)

1/2 cup vinegar
1/2 cup extra virgin olive oil
1 tablespoon green pepper, grated
1 tablespoon red pepper, grated
1 tablespoon fresh parsley, chopped
1 tablespoon dry mustard
1 tablespoon sugar
1/2 teaspoon salt
1/2 teaspoon paprika
1/8 teaspoon cayenne pepper
1/8 teaspoon pepper

1. Combine all ingredients in a sealable bowl, jar or serving carafe.

2. Chill vinaigrette at least two hours, overnight if possible.

3. Serve with cold meats, salads or vegetable asparagus.

Spiced Vinegar Veggies
(White Vinegar)

1/2 cup vinegar
1/2 cup water
1/4 cup cauliflower
1/4 cup broccoli
1/4 cup carrots
1/4 teaspoon dried thyme
1/8 teaspoon salt

1. Rinse vegetables and cut into bite-sized pieces.

2. Place vegetables in a large frying pan and add vinegar and water; blanch.

3. Add salt and dried thyme.

4. Refrigerate 3 days before serving.

Spiced Vinegar Mushrooms
(Apple Cider Vinegar)

1/2 cup vinegar
1 pound mushrooms, fresh not canned
3 cloves garlic, peeled and chopped
1 tablespoon virgin olive oil
1 tablespoon ginger
1 teaspoon soy sauce
1 teaspoon hot pepper sauce

1. Blanch mushrooms in boiling water for 2 minutes; drain and pat dry.

2. Mix everything in a jar with a tight fitting lid.

3. Refrigerate overnight.

4. Served alone or on spinach leaves.

Vinegar and Onions
(White Vinegar)

1/2 cup vinegar
1/2 cup water
3 tablespoons sugar
1 teaspoon salt, plus extra for sprinkling onion layer
1 pound tiny pearl onions
4 garlic cloves
1/2 teaspoon peppercorns

1. Wash tiny pearl onions; peel and blanch.

2. Lay onions out on a plate or cookie sheet and sprinkle with a thin layer of salt; set overnight.

3. In the morning, rinse salt from onions.

4. In a small bowl, combine vinegar, water, sugar and 1 teaspoon salt to make vinegar marinate.

5. Place onions in a pan and pour vinegar marinate over onions, just enough to cover them.

6. Add minced garlic and peppercorns and bring to a boil; boil until onions are tender; serve warm.

Beets
(White Vinegar)

1/2 cup vinegar
1/2 cup water
1/2 teaspoon salt
3 tablespoons sugar
3 fresh beets (or canned), cooked

1. Heat vinegar, water, salt and sugar over medium heat; bring to a boil.

2. Pour vinegar marinade over sliced beets.

3. Refrigerate for 24 hours before serving.

Crunchy Pickles
(White Vinegar)

1/3 cup vinegar
10-12 small cucumbers
1/3 cup kosher salt
1/3 cup fresh dill, chopped
1/2 teaspoon pickling spice
2 quarts water
2 garlic cloves, cut in half

1. In a glass container with a tight fitting lid, place washed cucumbers, dill, pickling spice and garlic pieces.

2. Pour vinegar, water and salt in a large saucepan or pot and boil for 3-4 minutes.

3. Pour hot vinegar solution over cucumbers in jar and replace lid.

4. Allow to set on countertop overnight.

5. Place jar in refrigerator to store; will last for several weeks.

Tangy Oriental Vegetable Dip
(Apple Cider Vinegar)

1/3 cup vinegar
1/2 cup plum jelly
1/3 cup applesauce
1 teaspoon brown sugar

1. Combine all ingredients together in a small bowl.

2. Serve with celery, carrots, cauliflower, broccoli, cherry tomatoes or other vegetable favorites.

Cooking Fish
(Apple Cider Vinegar)

Add a tangy zip to deep-fried battered fish.

vinegar, undiluted
spray bottle

1. After deep frying fish, remove from cooking oil and immediately spray with vinegar.

Vinegar Marinade for Meats
(Apple Cider Vinegar)

1 quart vinegar
2-3 red peppers
2 tablespoons brown sugar
1 onion, grated
1 tablespoon celery seed
1 tablespoon dry mustard
1 teaspoon pepper
1 teaspoon turmeric
1/2 teaspoon salt

1. Combine all ingredients together and place in a jar or plastic bottle; close lid.

2. Let age in a pantry or refrigerator for 3 weeks.

3. When ready to use, add 2-3 tablespoons to a stew, or sprinkle on meats prior to cooking.

Better Hot Dogs
(White Vinegar)

1 tablespoon vinegar

1. Add vinegar to water as you boil hot dots for better taste; pierce hot dogs before boiling and they will contain less fat and calories.

Baked Chicken
(Apple Cider Vinegar)

2 cups vinegar
4 chicken breasts
1 onion, finely chopped
1/4 cup olive oil
1/8 cup fresh thyme
2 tablespoons lemon juice
3 cloves garlic, minced
1 tablespoon sugar
2 tablespoons butter
1/2 teaspoon salt
ground pepper

1. In a frying pan, melt butter; add onions and cook over medium heat until onions are soft. Remove from heat.

2. Place chicken in a large bowl.

3. Add vinegar, olive oil, thyme, garlic, sugar, lemon juice, cooked onions, salt and pepper.

4. Cover bowl with plastic wrap and refrigerate 4 hours.

5. Preheat oven to 350°.

6. In a baking dish, arrange chicken breasts and pour vinegar marinade on top.

7. Bake for at least 1 hour, checking for doneness.

Vinegar Nut Pie Crust
(White Vinegar)

1 tablespoon vinegar
1/2 cup butter
3/4 cup flour
3/4 cup oatmeal
1/2 cup ground nuts (walnuts, pecans, etc.)
2 tablespoons sugar

1. Melt butter in a pie pan, and swirl around, being sure to "butter" entire pan.

2. Combine flour, oatmeal, ground nuts, sugar and vinegar in a small bowl.

3. Add flour mixture to buttered pie pan.

4. Gently press dough into pan.

5. Bake at 350° for 15-20 minutes; remove from oven and allow to cool completely.

6. Fill with favorite fruit filling.

Mint Sauce
(Apple Cider Vinegar)

1 cup vinegar
2 cups fresh mint leaves
2 tablespoons honey

1. Combine all ingredients in a blender.

2. This delicious mint sauce is wonderful served with lamb and peas, or as a dipping sauce.

Cherry-Pineapple Vinegar Cake
(White Vinegar)

3 tablespoons vinegar
1 cup whole milk
3/4 cup brown sugar
1 teaspoon baking soda
1 teaspoon allspice
3/4 pound flour
3/4 cup butter
1/2 pound candied cherries
1/2 pound candied pineapple

1. In a small bowl, combine vinegar and milk.

2. Add baking soda to milk mixture and stir vigorously; set aside.

3. In a mixing bowl, cream butter, sugar and flour together.

4. Add fruit and allspice to butter mixture.

5. Once combined, carefully fold in the milk and vinegar mixture and beat.

6. Bake in a greased pan at 350° for 1 hour, or until cake springs back when lightly touched.

7. Enjoy plain, or top with whipped cream and fresh fruit.

Peanut Butter Fudge
(White Vinegar)

1 tablespoon vinegar
3 1/2 cups sugar
1-12 ounce can evaporated milk
1/2 cup butter
1/4 cup corn syrup
3 cups peanut butter
1 cup marshmallow cream

1. Line a 9" x 13" pan lined with aluminum foil.

2. In a large saucepan, combine sugar, milk, butter, corn syrup and vinegar.

3. Cook over medium heat, stirring constantly, until mixture comes to a rolling boil.

4. Stir while boiling for 5 minutes; remove from heat.

5. Add peanut butter and marshmallow cream, stir until smooth; pour into prepared baking dish.

6. Allow to cool completely; cut into 1" squares.

Herbal Vinegar: Ginger
(Apple Cider Vinegar)
Try this accompaniment with oriental dishes

2 cups vinegar
1 teaspoon grated ginger

1. Pour vinegar into a glass jar or bottle with tight fitting lid.

2. Add grated ginger and seal jar tightly.

3. Set for 2- 4 weeks before using; swirl jar throughout 2-4 week period to incorporate flavors.

Vinegar Taffy
(White Vinegar)

3 tablespoons vinegar
2 cups sugar
1 tablespoon butter
1 teaspoon vanilla extract
1/2 cup water

1. Combine vinegar, sugar and water; boil to the hard ball stage.

2. Add butter and vanilla, and pour onto a greased plate or countertop.

3. When cool enough to touch, but still hot, begin to knead the taffy with buttered hands.

4. When taffy lightens in color and begins to firm, cut it into small, bite-sized pieces and wrap in waxed paper.

These flavored vinegars are a wonderful accompaniment to salads, meats, fruits and vegetables, as well as a simple and delicious way to further incorporate vinegar into your culinary world.

Herbal Vinegar: Garlic Vinegar
(Apple Cider Vinegar)

2 cups vinegar
4 garlic cloves

1. Pour vinegar into a jar with a tight sealing lid.

2. Add minced garlic and seal jar tightly.

3. Allow to set for at least one week.

Herbal Vinegar: Bay
(Apple Cider Vinegar)

This herbal vinegar is excellent with meats and pasta sauces.

2 cups vinegar
1/4 cup bay leaves, torn or crushed

1. Pour vinegar into a glass jar or bottle with tight fitting lid.

2. Add torn bay leaves and seal jar tightly.

3. Set for 2-4 weeks before using; swirl jar throughout 2-4 week period to incorporate flavors.

4. Herbal bay vinegar can be used as-is, or by straining out the bay leaves first, according to your own personal preference.

Herbal Vinegar: Horseradish
(Apple Cider Vinegar)

Try horseradish vinegar on cuts of beef or even your morning eggs for a little added zip.

2 cups vinegar
1 tablespoon horseradish, grated
2 cloves garlic, minced

1. Pour vinegar into a glass jar or bottle with tight fitting lid.

2. Add grated horseradish and minced garlic and seal jar tightly.

3. Set for 2 - 4 weeks before using; swirl jar throughout 2 – 4 week period to incorporate flavors.

Fortified Vinegars

These choice vinegars combine the nutritional value of a variety of fruits and vegetables with the rich goodness of vinegar. To make your own fortified vinegar, simply choose a favorite combination of fruits or vegetables (or both), and puree it in a blender along with a bit of apple cider vinegar. You can follow one of the formulas below, or concoct your own fortified vinegar adding your own favorite blend of spices and herbs. By making your own fortified vinegar, you can control the intensity of the flavor by adding more or less vinegar, or additional herbs and spices.

Fortified vinegars are excellent to use as marinades, salad dressings or flavorful dips.

Fortified Vinegars: Apple and Honey
(Apple Cider Vinegar)

Apple and honey vinegar is rich in calcium, beta carotene, carotenoids, chlorophyll, fiber, folacin, fructose, glucose, glycine, lecithin, lysine, pectin, niacin, selenium, sorbitol, sucrose, thiamin, tryptophan and zinc.

1 cup vinegar
1/2 cup honey
4 tart apples

1. Cut apples into large chunks and place in a blender; puree apples.

2. Add vinegar and honey.

3. Try this vinegar to over fresh fruit; use a tablespoon or two of this vinegar, then sprinkle with 1/2 teaspoon each of cinnamon and nutmeg.

Fortified Vinegar: Garlic
(Apple Cider Vinegar)

Garlic vinegar is very high in ascorbic acid, calcium, beta carotene, copper, fiber, glycine, lysine, niacin, riboflavin, selenium and thiamin.

1 cup vinegar
1/2 cup honey
4 tart apples, cut into chunks
1/2 cup oil
1/2 teaspoon salt
2 teaspoons sugar
2 teaspoons dry mustard
8 garlic bulbs, minced

1. Bake garlic in the oven at 200° until tender.

2. Place apple chunks in blender; puree apples, vinegar, honey, oil, salt, sugar and dry mustard.

3. Peel away outer skin of the garlic and squeeze the garlic paste into the blender.

4. Strain vinegar through a sieve to remove any seeds or lumps.

5. Enjoy over vegetables or a favorite beef entrée.

Fortified Vinegar: Mustard-Kale
(Apple Cider Vinegar)

Rich in antioxidants, beta carotene and fiber.

1 cup vinegar
1/4 water
2 cups kale
2 tablespoon

1. Combine all ingredients in a blender.

2. Use as a side accompaniment to vegetables.

Fortified Vinegar: Blueberry
(Apple Cider Vinegar)

This vinegar is rich in antioxidants, pectin, ascorbic acid, calcium, glucose, fructose, lysine, niacin, selenium, sorbitol, sucrose, thiamin, tryptophan and zinc. Try this concoction over fresh desserts.

1 cup vinegar
1/3 cup honey
4 tart apples, cut into chunks
2 cups blueberries
1/8 cup water
1 tablespoon lemon juice

1. Puree apples with vinegar and honey.

2. Add blueberries, water and lemon juice.

3. Strain vinegar through a sieve to remove any seeds or lumps.

Fortified Vinegar: Cucumber-Onion
(Apple Cider Vinegar)

Cucumber-onion vinegar is high in ascorbic acid, calcium, beta carotene, fiber, lysine, niacin, pectin, riboflavin, selenium and sulfur.

1 cup vinegar
1/2 cup onion, chopped
2 large cucumbers

1. Cut cucumber into chunks and place in the blender, peeling included.

2. Add onion and vinegar and blend together.

3. Great to use on vegetables or sliced fruit.

Fortified Vinegar: Cucumber-Celery
(Apple Cider Vinegar)

Rich in calcium, beta carotene, choline, copper, coumarin, beta elemene, glycine, histidine, iron, lysine, riboflavin, tryptophan, tyrosine, fluorine, selenium, beta sitosterol, thiamin.

1 cup vinegar
1 cup water
2 cups celery
1 large cucumber, cut into chunks
1/2 teaspoon salt

1. Puree cucumbers with rest of ingredients.

2. Blend together.

Plum – Blackberry Vinegar
(Apple Cider Vinegar)

2 cups vinegar
1/2 cup plums, peeled and mashed
1/2 cup blackberries, mashed
1/2 cup sugar

1. Rinse blackberries and mash well; peel and mash plumbs.

2. Pour vinegar into a glass carafe and add blackberries and plumbs. Refrigerate for 5 days.

3. Take vinegar and fruit combination and run thru a sieve, removing blackberry seeds.

4. Place plumb-blackberry vinegar on stove top and bring to a boil.

5. Add sugar and simmer until all the sugar has dissolved; cool completely.

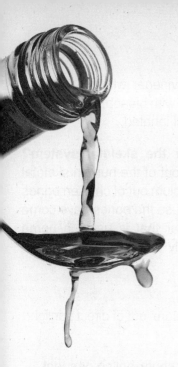

Chapter Nine

Frequently Asked Questions

Can white vinegar be substituted for apple cider vinegar?
White and apple cider vinegar may be substituted for each other, although one may be more useful than another in a particular situation.

Does vinegar expire or "go bad?"
Commercially produced vinegar has an indefinite shelf life. But, in actuality, vinegar can "go bad." If vinegar comes into contact with air for a long period of time, much of its chemical composition can breakdown and lose essential nutrients. If vinegar develops a rotten smell, the vinegar should be discarded and not used.

What is "Mother?"
Mother is a natural substance (cellulose) in vinegar that is derived from harmless vinegar bacteria. Most store bought vinegar has been pasteurized which keeps mother from forming while it is sitting on the shelf. If you notice mother forming in vinegar, simply strain it out.

Does vinegar contain fat or calories?
Vinegar contains about 3 calories in a tablespoon and is fat free.

Can vinegar be mixed with bleach?

Care should be taken not to combine vinegar with bleach. The high acid level in vinegar, in combination with bleach, can produce a harmful gas that could be dangerous if inhaled.

Is vinegar consumption harmful for the skeletal system?

It is a myth that vinegar draws calcium out of the human skeletal system. Although vinegar does draw calcium out of chicken bones to help make broth and soups, it is because the bones have come into direct contact with vinegar. Vinegar that is used in home remedies and recipes is taken internally and does not come in direct contact with bones.

Where should I store vinegar?

It is best to store vinegar at room temperature, out of direct sunlight.

Can I purchase vinegar in bulk?

To purchase large quantities of vinegar, check online or speak with the manager of your local grocery store.

Can using vinegar interact with prescription medication?

As with any home remedy, be sure and contact your health care provider prior to beginning any health regimen using vinegar.

Can I make my own vinegar?

Yes, you can make your own vinegar. For more information, check out *The Vinegar Book* and *The Vinegar Book II* on how to begin.

Is vinegar gluten free?

Some vinegars are gluten free, and others are not. Be sure and check the bottle labeling to find out if your particular vinegar contains gluten.

What is the difference between distilled vinegar and white vinegar?

Generally speaking, people use the terms "distilled vinegar" and "white vinegar" interchangeably. Technically, there are subtle differences in chemical makeup between the two, and distilled vinegar has been purified more than white vinegar.

Additional Publications
By Emily Thacker

Additional books by Emily Thacker can be ordered
using the attached order form at the back of this book,
or by visiting our website at
http://www.jamesdirect.com

THE VINEGAR BOOK

Everyone loves vinegar! Its piquant bite blends well with
an endless number of other foods. It tenderizes, enhances and
preserves foods. More importantly, vinegar is a terrific germ killer.
It is active against bacteria, viruses, molds and fungus. This safe,
healing food can be found all across the world in many forms and
flavors.

It is the traveler's friend, as it helps to prevent the system
upsets that often plague tourists. Research has shown it to
be effective in killing flu germs. It is also known for its anti-itch
properties and its muscle soothing abilities.

Vinegar's long history as a panacea for the aches and pains
of this world is respected in many cultures and places. Anyone
who is serious about natural healing, old time remedies or folk
medicine *must* have this book!

THE VINEGAR BOOK II

This delightful addition takes you through the year, with a vinegar use for each day. Twelve chapters, one for each month, combine the 365 vinegar based hints with explanations of how vinegar is made, why it is so healthful and how it has been used down through thousands of years.

You will learn of vinegar's uses in cooking and preserving and about its value is preventing diseases. This includes its importance in fighting cancer and arthritis, as well as how vinegar can be used to actually "cook" protein, such as fish.

This book also contains easy directions for making fruit, vegetable and herbal vinegars. Learn how to begin with apple cider vinegar and add valerian as a sleep aid, bay leaves to sharpen the memory or gota kola to fight stress. You will also find a recipe for making imitation balsamic vinegar that rivals the expensive varieties for taste and usefulness!

VINEGAR HOME GUIDE

Vinegar contains a host of germ fighting components, having both antibiotic and antiseptic properties. It has the ability to actually kill mold and mildew spores. And, it can contain natural tannins which help to preserve foods.

Vinegar is a completely biodegradable product nature can easily break it down into components that feed and nurture plant life. This makes it superior to chemical cleaners that poison the soil today and remain in it and destroy plant life for many years.

This helpful book is packed full of ways to use vinegar around the home, in the garden, on pets and to clean the car, boat or camper. You will want to use vinegar in your humidifier, to strip wallpaper, repair wood scratches kill mold on refrigerator and freezer gaskets and to make both play-clay and mouthwashes.

To order use the handy order form in the back of this book,
or online at **http://www.jamesdirect.com**

VINEGAR AND TEA

Green tea is soothing to the body and healing for the spirit. Research continues to add to the list of healing properties of green tea. It is a safe, tasty way to lose weight and improve health.

For years tea has been used to improve health and vitality. Studies and detailed analysis show that the type of caffeine in tea is less likely to cause the irritating, jittery symptoms of coffee and other caffeine containing substances. Tea is often considered a calming liquid that brings a sense of well being and serenity.

The *Vinegar & Tea* book describes the way tea is produced and grown and explains which kinds may be perfect for you. It covers delicate white teas, healing green ones and bold black blends. It will guide you in choosing the perfect tea to heal illnesses or soothe a troubled spirit.

VINEGAR ANNIVERSARY

The Vinegar Anniversary Book blends the contents of Emily Thacker's four books on vinegar into one big book!

The original *Vinegar Book* details hundreds of old time healing remedies plus information on how to clean with vinegar. You will learn about the many different kinds of vinegar – from apple cider, wine, rice and malt to more exotic kinds such as banana and date.

The *Vinegar Book II* offers 365 vinegar uses to let you try a new one every day of the year.

The *Vinegar Home Guide* focuses on using vinegar for cleaning and disinfecting around the home, yard and garden.

The *Vinegar Diet Book* brings the healthy goodness of vinegar to the table in an exciting, safe way to easily control weight. It offers wholesome, nourishing insight into managing what you eat. You will find this is the easiest, most foolproof diet plan you have ever tried!

THE CINNAMON BOOK

Some consider cinnamon the king of "Anti"s. Scientific research studies have shown that cinnamon is rich in natural healing properties making it anti-inflammatory, anti-septic, anti-microbial, anti-oxidant, anti-clotting, anti-tumor, anti-parasitic and anti-fungal! All this works to make cinnamon one of the most potent natural health remedies around!

Not only is this amazing spice excellent for better health, but also equally amazing when used for beauty purposes. It also can rid the home of insects, works as a fragrant aromatic, and can dye fabrics. Cinnamon is healthy in the diet, and as we already know, tastes delicious!

The Cinnamon Book offers 208 pages of cinnamon home remedies, health and beauty regimens, around-the-home uses and of course, a few wonderful recipes!

THE HONEY BOOK

Research studies have shown that honey possesses unique and remarkable nutrients that bring healing to the body effectively and naturally, without harmful side effects that occur with so many pharmaceutical medications. Honey is an all-natural, inexpensive and readily-available alternative to treat the body's ailments.

Honey contains powerful antibacterial and antimicrobial qualities that disinfect open cuts, wounds and bacterial infections. Honey is also excellent for treating fatigue, arthritis and joint pains, digestion problems and respiratory ailments — just to name a few!

The Honey Book is 208 pages of natural home remedies, research and recipes for putting honey to use immediately against some of your most bothersome health issues and conditions.

To order use the handy order form in the back of this book, or online at **http://www.jamesdirect.com**

GARLIC: NATURE'S NATURAL COMPANION

This volume is a celebration of the miraculous healing powers of garlic! From earliest times garlic's ability to kill germs and heal sickness has been recognized. It has been used as an amulet to frighten away vampires and combined with vinegar to make the Thieves' Vinegar that reputedly offered protection from the plague.

Garlic grows almost everywhere, from the cold of Siberia and Tibet to the warmth of the Mediterranean and sunny California. Much of the world's supply is grown in China, who ships it out by the ton. It comes in tiny, intense, almost bitter bulbs to large elephant garlic bulbs.

The wonder of this versatile food is celebrated in festivals and fairs. Cook offs feature it in surprising recopies. Garlic is truly one of the healthiest, most widely used healing foods on the planet!

THE MAGIC OF BAKING SODA

Do you keep your baking soda in the refrigerator or in the medicine cabinet? Or, perhaps you keep it with your laundry or cleaning supplies? You will want to keep it in your kitchen, medicine cabinet and with your cleaning and laundry supplies.

Baking soda is a naturally occurring substance that is kind to the environment. It is used to soothe allergies, exactly the opposite of many harsh chemical cleaning supplies.

Whether it is to soothe an acid stomach or the itching of rashes, baking soda is a must-have for the medicine cabinet. It is used in hospitals to protect the kidneys from intravenous dyes used in CT scans and to assist in dialysis treatments. Make sure you are getting all the benefits possible from this inexpensive substance you already have in your home.

THE HYDROGEN PEROXIDE BOOK

This book discovers the unique qualities of hydrogen peroxide as both a valuable home remedy and an incredible cleaning resource.

Hydrogen peroxide has a long history of medicinal use. It is well know for its ability to cleanse and disinfect wounds, promote rapid healing, and prevent infection. It is used in hospitals, nursing homes and child care facilities nationwide.

Its cleaning abilities are boundless, working to purify water, kill bacteria and sterilize everything from kitchens to bathrooms.

It is also an amazing health and beauty aid, working well on hair and skin.

Hydrogen peroxide even safely works wonders in the garden!

EMILY'S DISASTER GUIDE OF
NATURAL REMEDIES

Emily's Disaster Guide of Natural Remedies is a unique guide written to highlight some of the many threats we face, both natural and manmade, and ways to prepare and protect your family.

Included in this guide is an overview of current events and the state our communities are in. You will also find a list of infectious diseases and conditions, along with possible treatments.

PLUS each book contains its own Emergency Preparedness Checklist and Emergency Family Plan to help your family prepare for any emergency.

To order use the handy order form in the back of this book, or online at **http://www.jamesdirect.com**

Index

✂ please cut here

Use this coupon to order "The Vinegar Formula Guide" for a friend or family member -- or copy the ordering information onto a plain piece of paper and mail to:

The Vinegar Formula Guide
Dept. VF134
PO Box 980
Hartville, Ohio 44632

Preferred Customer Reorder Form

Order this...	If you want a book on...	Cost...	Number of Copies...
Garlic: Nature's Natural Companion	Exciting scientific research on garlic's ability to promote good health. Find out for yourself why garlic has the reputation of being able to heal almost magically! Newest in Emily's series of natural heath books!	$9.95	
Amish Gardening Secrets	You too can learn the special gardening secrets the Amish use to produce huge tomato plants and bountiful harvests. Information packed 800-plus collection for you to tinker with and enjoy.	$9.95	
The Vinegar Home Guide	Learn how to clean and freshen with natural, environmentally-safe vinegar in the house, garden and laundry. Plus, delicious home-style recipes!	$9.95	
Emily's Disaster Guide of Natural Remedies	Emily's new guide to infectious diseases & their threat on our health. What happens if we can't get to the pharmacy – or the shelves are empty, *what then?* What if the electricity goes out – and stays out? What if my neighborhood was quarantined? How would I feed my family? Handle first aid? 208 page book!	$9.95	

Any combination of the above $9.95 items qualifies for the following discounts...

| | **Total NUMBER of $9.95 items** | |

Order any 2 items for: **$15.95**

Order any 3 items for: **$19.95**

Order any 4 items for: **$24.95**

Order any 5 items for: **$29.95**

Order any 6 items for: **$34.95** and receive 7th item FREE

Any additional items for: **$5 each**

FEATURED SELECTIONS

		Total COST of $9.95 items	
The Magic of Baking Soda	*Plain Old Baking Soda A Drugstore in A Box?* Doctors & researchers have discovered baking soda has amazing healing properties! Over 600 health & Household Hints. *Great Recipes Too!*	$12.95	
The Vinegar Anniversary Book	Completely updated with the latest research and brand new remedies and uses for apple cider vinegar. Handsome coffee table collector's edition you'll be proud to display. **Big 208-page book!**	$12.95	
Vinegar Formula Guide	This one-of-a-kind, ground breaking book gives you exact formulas and measurements for ALL of your vinegar applications! In it you'll find step-by-step, easy-to-use instructions for home health remedies, cleaning projects and more!	$19.95	
The Honey Book	Amazing Honey Remedies to relieve arthritis pain, kill germs, heal infection and much more!	$19.95	
The Magic of Hydrogen Peroxide	An Ounce of Hydrogen Peroxide is worth a Pound of Cure! Hundreds of health cures, household uses & home remedy uses for hydrogen peroxide contained in this breakthrough volume.	$19.95	

Order any 2 or more Featured Selections for only $10 each...

	Postage & Handling	$3.98*
	TOTAL	

*** Shipping of 10 or more books = $6.96**

90-Day Money-Back Guarantee

Please rush me the items marked above. I understand that I must be completely satisfied or I can return any item within 90 days with proof of purchase for a full and prompt refund of my purchase price.

I am enclosing $_____ by: ❑ Check ❑ Money Order (Make checks payable to James Direct Inc)

Charge my credit card Signature _____

Card No. _____ Exp. Date _____

Name _____ Address _____

City _____ State_____ Zip _____

Telephone Number (_____) _____

❑ Yes! I'd like to know about freebies, specials and new products before they are nationally advertised. My email address is: _____

VISA MasterCard Discover AMEX

Mail To: **James Direct Inc.** • PO Box 980, Dept. A1347 • Hartville, Ohio 44632
Customer Service (330) 877-0800 • *http://www.jamesdirect.com*

GARLIC: NATURE'S NATURAL COMPANION
Explore the very latest studies and new remedies using garlic to help with cholesterol, blood pressure, asthma, arthritis, digestive disorders, bacteria, cold and flu symptoms, and MUCH MORE! Amazing cancer studies!

- -

AMISH GARDENING SECRETS
There's something for everyone in *Amish Gardening Secrets*. This BIG collection contains over 800 gardening hints, suggestions, time savers and tonics that have been passed down over the years in Amish communities and elsewhere.

- -

THE VINEGAR HOME GUIDE
Emily Thacker presents her second volume of hundreds of all-new vinegar tips. Use versatile vinegar to add a low-sodium zap of flavor to your cooking, as well as getting your house "white-glove" clean for just pennies. Plus, safe and easy tips on shining and polishing brass, copper & pewter and removing stubborn stains & static cling in your laundry!

- -

EMILY'S DISASTER GUIDE OF NATURAL REMEDIES
Emily's most important book yet! If large groups of the population become sick at the same time, the medical services in this country will become stressed to capacity. *What then?* We will all need to know what to do! Over 307 natural cures, preventatives, cure-alls and ways to prepare to naturally treat & prevent infectious disease.

- -

THE MAGIC OF BAKING SODA
We all know baking soda works like magic around the house. It cleans, deodorizes & works wonders in the kitchen and in the garden. But did you know it's an effective remedy for allergies, bladder infection, heart disorders… *and MORE!*

- -

THE VINEGAR ANNIVERSARY BOOK
Handsome coffee table edition and brand new information on Mother Nature's Secret Weapon – apple cider vinegar!

- -

VINEGAR FORMULA GUIDE
Studies have shown vinegar to be effective at not only cleaning and disinfecting, but also as a natural home remedy for conditions such as lowering cholesterol, fighting disease, easing arthritis, improving circulation and more! Now learn the exact formulas and measurements for EACH home remedy and cleaning project in a concise, easy-to-read format! No more guess-work!

- -

THE HONEY BOOK
Each page is packed with healing home remedies and ways to use honey to heal wounds, fight tooth decay, treat burns, fight fatigue, restore energy, ease coughs and even make cancer-fighting drugs more effective. Great recipes too!

- -

THE MAGIC OF HYDROGEN PEROXIDE
Hundreds of health cures & home remedy uses for hydrogen peroxide. You'll be amazed to see how a little hydrogen peroxide mixed with a pinch of this or that from your cupboard can do everything from relieving chronic pain to making age spots go away! Easy household cleaning formulas too!

* Each Book has its own FREE Bonus!